DEATH BENEFITS

DEATH BENEFITS

How Losing a Parent Can
Change an Adult's Life—
For the Better

Jeanne Safer, Ph.D.

BASIC
B
BOOKS

A Member of the Perseus Books Group
New York

Books published by Basic Books are available at special discounts for bulk purchases in the United States by corporations, institutions, and other organizations. For more information, please contact the Special Markets Department at the Perseus Books Group, 2300 Chestnut Street, Suite 200, Philadelphia, PA 19103, or call (800) 255-1514, or e-mail special.markets@perseusbooks.com.

Designed by Timm Bryson
Set in 11 point Adobe Caslon

Library of Congress Cataloging-in-Publication Data
Safer, Jeanne.
Death benefits : how losing a parent can change an adult's life—for the better / Jeanne Safer.
p. cm.
Includes bibliographical references and index.
ISBN 978-0-465-07211-8
1. Death—Social aspects. 2. Parents—Death—Psychological aspects. 3. Adult children—Psychology. I. Title.
HQ1073.S24 2008
155.9'37—dc22

2007046573

10 9 8 7 6 5 4 3 2 1

For Linda Marshall

Perhaps nobody is completely grown-up until both his parents are dead.

—AUBERON WAUGH, *Will This Do?* (1991)

Contents

PART III

ORPHANS' BENEFITS:
SEEING PARENTS WITH NEW EYES

PART IV

IN MORTE VERITAS:
THE INSIGHTS DEATH BRINGS

INTRODUCTION

Life After Death

‿〰‿

The death of your parents can be the best thing that ever happens to you.

I know it sounds shocking—almost sacrilegious—to assert that one of the most devastating losses you suffer in adulthood could turn out to be your greatest gain. What about the Fifth Commandment, "Honor Thy Father and Thy Mother"? What about common decency and respect for the dead?

What about devotion?

Losing a parent almost always causes pain and sorrow; these are the wages of love. Their deaths sever the first and deepest ties of our lives and make us uncomfortably mindful that we're next in line. The world seems impoverished when a beloved parent, however flawed, no longer inhabits it; part of us dies with him or her. If the parent suffered or the child was burdened with caretaking responsibilities at the end, relief mingles with grief, and anyone who had a truly terrible mother or father—one who was brutal, neglectful, or hateful—naturally feels liberated finally to be out of harm's way. Still, even in these cases death hardly seems cause for celebration.

But the premise of this book is exactly that: I have found that the death of a parent—any parent—can set us free. It offers us our last, best chance to become our truest, deepest selves. It creates unique opportunities for growth—possibilities unimaginable before and not available by any other means. Nothing else in adult life has so much unrecognized potential to help us become more fulfilled human beings—wiser, more mature, more open, less afraid.

~ೋ~

Parent loss is the most potent catalyst for change in middle age, the time in life at which most people undergo it. Although 5 percent of the population loses a mother or father every year, few of us are psychologically prepared for the experience. *Death Benefits* is the handbook for exploring the uncharted territory we enter when a parent leaves us, in both senses, alone—and on the verge of previously inconceivable positive changes in every aspect of our lives.

I know about death benefits because I have experienced them. I have also witnessed remarkable changes in my patients who have lost their parents. Though I am a trained psychotherapist who has been in practice for thirty-five years, and who has spent many years in psychotherapy myself, only my mother's death opened my eyes and allowed me to heal certain wounds. Then I was able to understand and to alter ways of thinking and feeling I never believed I could change. My intention is to illuminate the process I went through, to document and interpret the thoughts and feelings, memories, dreams, and insights I had as I struggled to understand my relationship with this formidable woman, who died three years ago at the age of ninety-two—and who took everything in my power to comprehend. I hope that my discoveries provide a new, systematic, and comprehensive model for others to follow.

I also interviewed sixty insightful and inspiring midlife men and women who discovered death benefits in their own lives—physically, mentally, and spiritually. Some changed in ways so subtle that nobody else noticed, and others literally looked and acted like different people. My goal is to make the metamorphosis I, my patients, and my interview subjects underwent available to others who want to emerge from mourning with enriched lives.

Among the people you will meet whom orphanhood transformed are these:

- A thirty-eight-year-old publicist whose heart belonged to her autocratic and possessive daddy and who finally fell in love and married when he died;
- A forty-nine-year-old repressed teacher who discovered her true vocation as an actress and came to passionate life on stage after she lost her self-involved, demanding mother;
- A fifty-five-year-old historian whose luminous, consoling dream of his dead mother's loving arms helped him rediscover his childhood religious faith.

Although many midlife adults experience death benefits, too few feel comfortable admitting that they have done so, and even fewer have any idea how to actively bring them about, let alone plan for them. Don't leave something so important, precious, and urgent to chance. Death benefits take serious effort to achieve, but with the proper tools they are now available to every adult who loses a parent.

"Profiting" from a parent's death is not incompatible with grief and loss; in fact, mourning is a prerequisite. Having unfinished business (anger, guilt, disappointment) with that parent—or parent surrogate—need not prevent you from having a better life as a result of their demise; finishing some of that business is one of the biggest positive consequences you can achieve, and one of the most common.

Even though we cannot choose our parents or alter our past relationship with them, we can have conscious input into which aspects of them we embody after they are gone: a task we can only undertake in what I call the Deathspace, the new perspective that opens up in the wake of their loss. We can also go unimpeded for the first time in new directions in love, in work, and in understanding. Here you will find personal and professional guidance for an enterprise that most people undertake haphazardly and without awareness.

Death Benefits is about self-transformation in later life and how to employ critical, even intensely painful life experiences to achieve the insights that make it happen. It challenges the conventional wisdom that fundamental change is only for the young, and that loss must simply be endured, denied, or overcome.

One of the many advantages of the perspective death affords you is being able to see your parent as a person and a peer, often with new empathy and sympathy. You may discover, as many people do, that the posthumous relationship you create with a parent is more gratifying and three-dimensional than the relationship you had during the parent's lifetime. And you can start the process at any time; it will unfold and become ever richer as life goes on. Death benefits grow along with you.

Pursuing death benefits can and should be a conscious, systematic process. Much of the psychological work goes on at the deepest levels, but organized, repeated efforts, based on the interlocking series of practices, questions and actions that I followed and that are elaborated in the text, will help you succeed:

Four Practices to Cultivate Death Benefits

Motivate. Make a conscious decision to address and learn from your parent's death, investing time and energy in the project.

Anticipate. Give yourself permission to seek death benefits and identify your resistance to doing so.

Meditate. Cultivate a receptive stance. Think seriously about both the positive and negative impact your parent has had on your life, and the unfinished business between you.

Activate. Death benefits are available at any time, and evolve over time. Take these actions periodically to pursue them:

- Construct a narrative of your parent's history as objectively as possible;
- Conduct an inventory of your parent's character, determining what to keep and what to discard;
- Seek new experiences and relationships to support the changes you desire.

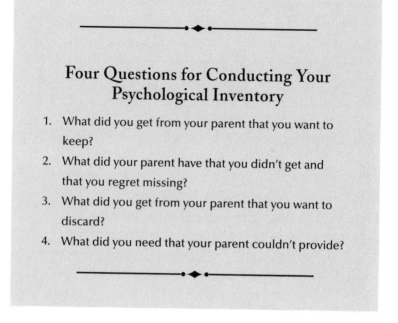

Four Questions for Conducting Your Psychological Inventory

1. What did you get from your parent that you want to keep?
2. What did your parent have that you didn't get and that you regret missing?
3. What did you get from your parent that you want to discard?
4. What did you need that your parent couldn't provide?

Death Benefits conveys a message of hope—that grievous losses can be the basis of insight and wisdom, and that the ultimate shape your life and your character take are to a large extent in your hands. There are always possibilities for growth and change, ever-expanding opportunities to reassess and reconstruct your relationship with deceased parents, and in so doing, with yourself and your world.

My goal is for death benefits to be taboo no longer but rather a part of every adult's inheritance. We speak of birthrights—let us also speak of deathrights. Although I believe that becoming an orphan is a major loss, no matter what your relationship with a parent was, I also believe that you can turn it into a major gain. I hope this book, and the stories in it, provide inspiration and guidance to make the years after bereavement the best years of your life.

PART I

DEATH CHANGES
EVERYTHING

CHAPTER I

My Death Benefit

(Autobiography)

❧

Red Is a Neutral

I feel less alone since my mother died. It is shocking and comforting to realize this. I think of her every day. I use her fifty-year-old KitchenAid coffee grinder and her Italian dishes, hand-painted with mushrooms. Her photograph, handsome and dramatic at age ninety, sits above my chair in my office. I look at the arrangement of paintings and ethnic textiles on my walls, the original way I dress—sometimes I notice the expressions on my face, the phrases or tones of voice I remember her using—and I see her reflection, probably more often than I did when she was alive. I speak of her frequently, usually with admiration; curiously, I never find myself speaking *to* her, even in dreams. But I have gradually and reluctantly come to know that something awful I was prone to when she was in the world, something utterly at odds with my forceful, even optimistic, nature is fading: a certain hopeless dread that comes over me, a steep descent into panic when I feel sick or helpless that I can't remember ever being free of. It would grieve her to be implicated. I know its diminished hold on me has to do with her absence.

Even though I am the person others turn to for sustenance and good advice—I was such a natural at it that I made it my profession—I have always been inconsolable. That I lacked what seems to be other people's birthright was my most shameful secret. My husband feels none of this, even when he had a cancer that could have been fatal; I've been more terrified of a cold. Happily, I could comfort him. No one could comfort me.

Only now, three years after her death at ninety-two, do I know why. I was bound to her by a loyalty so deeply buried that twenty years of therapy did not reveal it. She had to be the sole source of comfort, even though she was wrong for the job. I could not go elsewhere, and so I had to do without. A combination of love and desperation bound me to prop up her notion of herself as a mother. Though she genuinely tried to be one and sometimes succeeded, I had to protect us both from her frequent failures. As a result there was a cliff I could always fall off; there was no psychic safety net for me.

This knowledge has been dawning on me incrementally since she died; the secret was impenetrable before. Keeping it so was part of my unspoken mission, and that mission is accomplished. Her death lifted the information embargo and left me free to explore the sealed archive. Now that there is no one I have to sustain but me, I can let myself see the truth.

All my adult life I had noticed how easily distress can catapult me into bottomless terror, but I had never been able to figure out why, let alone do much about it. A subway stuck in a tunnel, a ring stuck on my finger, changes in my sensorium (intrusive noise, untoward physical experiences of illness)—things nobody likes but most people take in stride—tormented me and made me feel invaded. A claustrophobia-like sense that I can't stand to be in my own skin or in the situation another second rapidly sets in. As much as I hated and feared the inner abyss, it still yawned open periodically; this vulnerability was the only aspect of my emotional life where strenuous effort made few inroads. Despite everything else I have overcome, my failure to change the intensity of my reaction to certain kinds of adversity made me feel weak and helpless and fraudulent; a psychoanalyst incapable of penetrating the most wounded part of her own psyche is like an out-of-shape personal trainer.

My mother's death has done more to alleviate my anxiety than hypnosis, biofeedback, and meditation (all of which I've tried) combined. It galvanized me to try again, with a dramatically different attitude. Suddenly I found the will to confront my nightmare state, and this time my goal was nothing less than to limit its power over me. I vowed that I would spare no effort to avoid taking it to my own grave, which I seemed to be approaching at an accelerated rate because she was no longer there to shield me. As soon as she was gone I felt capable of facing the fear and finding its origins, even excited at the prospect. Then meanings and connections rushed to me with the force of revelation.

I primed myself for my exploration of my darkest recesses by looking for clues to our relationship in the fragments of my mother's history that I know; for someone so verbal, she told me surprisingly little about her early life, and I have no contact with the few members of her family who are still alive. When I went through her possessions, I found eloquent artifacts and a few letters she had written and received before I was born—as well as every one I ever wrote to her, collected in the box where they had been reposing since the 1960s. I also reconsidered my own memories and assumptions. I wanted to see things differently.

The first thing I did was look at her. The photograph in my office displays the quintessential "Esther" as she was in her last years. It is such an arresting physical presence that I find it hard to believe she's no longer alive. She lounges, her lustrous silver hair swinging over her face, on a tiger-printed throw, stroking the color-coordinated calico cat that became her companion and surrogate daughter. She wears pink cashmere with a long kaleidoscopic silk scarf draped around her neck, gold chains dangling with golden fish, a thrift-shop pink plastic bracelet dotted with rhinestones. Her subtly made-up face is not beautiful—she has a prominent nose and no cheekbones to speak of—but she has an allure more enduring than beauty—wit, instinctive elegance, and a style all her own; self-absorbed but not vain. She has arranged her face in a not entirely believable enigmatic smile, and she isn't looking at the camera.

My mother's striking persona, along with her physical magnetism and her inspired eye for personal as well as interior decoration, is the most compelling thing about her. It is also the key to her character, as much for what it conceals as for what it reveals. For sixty years I couldn't see past it.

Everybody—men, women, dogs—noticed Esther. She was flirtatious but never provocative; repairmen and mechanics were at her feet. The aplomb with which this untutored woman presented herself to the world was her most potent expression of will, her most enduring source of satisfaction. All her life, despite everything that happened to her, she had verve, fervor, and flair, as well as a pair of sensational legs that her daughter did not inherit. Neither breast cancer, nor adultery, nor the death of her son felled her. After my father died, she went back to work at age sixty-eight, traveled extensively, and lived alone by choice for the next twenty years. The way she moved and threw herself into everything that fascinated her expressed a vitality that not even the ravages of dementia could erode; she died with her personality intact. She danced and swam daily until her late eighties; only cognitive decline and a heart attack slowed her down at the very end. When I bought her sarong pants and three-inch-long beaded earrings for her ninetieth birthday, the saleswoman begged to meet her. Nobody else's mother looked like mine, and nobody believed she was only 5'2".

Her three tones of voice are as indelible as her presence: her laugh, her authoritative air, and, on some wretched occasions, her rageful coldness. I can still hear the sound of her laughter (she couldn't tell a joke, becoming helpless with mirth when she tried) and feel the deadly rejection, the screaming silence, when I disappointed her. But it was her voice of command that really defined her. It impressed me as much as it infuriated me—and this (my patients and my husband inform me) I did inherit. I always took her authoritativeness as gospel, even when I found out later that she had her facts, and often her feelings, wrong. "Remember, Jeanne," she used to tell me with the intonation she reserved for major pronouncements, as if expounding a Law of Nature, "red is a neutral." There was nothing whatsoever neutral about her. Nor was I the only one to whom she imparted this sacred principle; at her funeral, all her caretakers wore it in her honor.

For the longest time I felt drab and awkward around her. This was one of the many ways, I now know, that I maintained her in the starring role she needed. Not until my thirties, when I was a naturalized New Yorker, married, and established in my career, was my separate identity finally solid enough for me to incorporate elements of her style into what was becoming my own. Her signature color began to infiltrate my all-black wardrobe and spilled onto my floors and furniture over the years, first as an occasional accent, later as the avant-garde of a riot of other colors and patterns (we share a penchant for paisleys and animal prints). Like so many things, she turned out to be right about this. I also joined a Renaissance chorus, studied belly dance for years, and at age fifty-eight started working seriously with a swim coach—all variations on things she loved. Now no one would ever mistake me for anybody's daughter but hers, and I often hear the sweetest words in the English language, words she would be thrilled that I inspire: "Are you in the arts?"

But her many charms—as authentic and memorable as they are—were ultimately more impressive to strangers than to her near relations. She made an impression on everyone, but she never relied on anyone but me.

The Reluctant Mirror

After I looked at her photograph, I looked at her life, organizing it and laying out the narrative. Like a clinician examining a case history, I tried to see my mother as objectively and compassionately as possible, as I was only able to do when death permanently divided us. Who was she as a daughter, a wife, a mother, a woman? What were her demons, her flaws, her struggles, her triumphs? They were all part of my legacy. My goal was to expand my field of vision; I couldn't take a meaningful psychological inventory of her character until I understood it. Systematically constructing her biography was the prerequisite and foundation—my most critical tool for reaping death benefits.

My mother was one of four children of Russian Jewish immigrants to Cincinnati, Ohio, the baby by many years. Finances dictated that she alone of her artistically talented siblings be allowed to finish high school. A natural musician who played the piano by ear, she was offered a scholarship in voice by the local conservatory, which her devout, tyrannical father would not allow her to accept, deeming the vocation unsuitable for a respectable daughter of his. Her mother, whom she always wistfully called "Momma," did not intervene on her behalf.

I knew my maternal grandmother as an elderly woman, and she made surprisingly little impression on me. Though she must have had a certain fragile beauty in her youth, she seemed passive and beaten by then, in total contrast to her spirited youngest child, whom I had the feeling had always been her designated caretaker and confidante. My mother keenly regretted her own limited formal education and compensated by taking art and humanities courses for years. She would also make sure that I acquired what she was denied: an advanced degree and the economic independence that comes with it.

Families like hers had the aspiration that their boys become doctors and their girls marry one. She fulfilled this goal by finding a wry, introverted anesthesiologist beguiled by her energy and pizzazz, although his parents—two of the few people she never impressed—considered her beneath his station. She threw herself into the roles ordained for her, cooking, baking, entertaining, and having the requisite two babies, while living in a crowded apartment downstairs from the mother-in-law who despised her and refused to speak to her.

My mother's first child, my brother, Steven, was a major disappointment early on, with serious school and social problems. Out of shame, my father stubbornly refused to take him to a psychiatrist; my mother, repeating her own mother's pattern, never overrode his edict, and never forgave herself. I don't remember her as depressed—it would be difficult to detect in someone so active—but her expression in some of the photographs of her as a young wife shows signs of bewildered distress.

Around the time of Steven's birth, my father developed severe ulcerative colitis, the first of a lifetime of chronic illnesses that demoralized him and caused him to withdraw. Seven years later, when I was born, he was informed that his heart was so seriously damaged that he would undoubtedly die young—even though he actually survived thirty more years on what had to feel like borrowed time. When I was eleven, he spent three months in the hospital with peritonitis; my mother virtually moved into his room to attend him expertly.

The secure world she thought would be her refuge and the platform for her talents after the strictures of her childhood seemed to be collapsing. She had a son she could not mother (she never ceased alternatively blaming him and herself for the ruins of their relationship, and he died from complications of diabetes a year before she did, estranged from me as well as from her) and a husband terrified about his health and increasingly dissatisfied with his profession and their marriage. She was desperately seeking solace and affirmation, and she turned to me.

I was my mother's consolation and her prize—her project, her companion, her achievement, her mirror. Determining at my birth that I would be a writer and therefore needed a nom de plume, she gave me the exotic and masculine-sounding name "Gene"; my father, with no such agenda, insisted I be called the more feminine "Jeanne." She grudgingly admired my strong will and the "determined jaw" I was born with, which she saw as an indication that we were kindred spirits. Every possible talent and ability was lovingly, generously cultivated (including some I actually had, although I didn't fulfill the prime directive and begin to write professionally until my late forties). I became, to my mother's delight and relief, "unusual"—the student every teacher loved, the child upon whom she could lavish all her gifts and all her attention—her second chance.

With everything she gave me, my mother asked a great deal back, while denying she asked anything at all. The most taxing of her demands was paradoxical: I was to fulfill all her potential as well as my own, but we must always remain the center of each other's universe; I could do anything I wanted but leave. She protested repeatedly that she was too sophisticated for her conventional Midwestern hometown but felt betrayed when I eventually moved to New York City for good, though she clearly groomed me to do so. I never imagined, any more than she did, how much I sustained her. Her exterior belied it; my unspoken responsibility was to make sure nothing interfered with that image for either one of us.

In most situations my mother took charge with her red-is-a-neutral authority, but on close inspection I see there were gigantic gaps, which I noiselessly filled for her. She was a superb woman in a crisis, as long as it didn't threaten her inconsolable core. In times of calamity the delicate balance between my needs and my mother's collapsed. Then she had to obliterate me. At these moments—there were only a handful, but they were life-defining—I lost her completely as the guardian of my security.

The way my mother dealt with her miserable living situation, which with the rest of her travails must have pushed her endurance to the breaking point, was the first time this happened, and it shocks me still. Unable to insist that they move away from her in-laws' aegis to a home of their own, she made a suicide threat in front of me (I was six at the time) that had the effect of persuading my father to take action. I didn't find out until my twenties when she confessed to me that she considered it her only recourse; clearly I'd had to forget because the implications were so disturbing.

The problem, then and later, was not that she ignored my feelings or the impact of her actions on me when she felt trapped, but rather that she failed to consider me as a separate person altogether. I became her instrument and her prop, her ultimate accessory, without feelings of my own. That it might harm me to be used in this way could not enter her mind because our needs were identical; you can't damage your own reflection. As I got older I was expected to do far more than simply be there; I became her witness. If I protested or refused to do what she required of me, this fault line in my mother's character made her turn on me like a Fury, and I became her enemy. Because she couldn't bear to think of herself as failing me (unlike her own mother, she had to be a perfect one), she ended up accusing me of failing her.

My solution was to implement a form of evasive action so elegant that I never knew I was doing anything: I instinctively started protecting her by asserting emotional self-sufficiency precisely in the areas where she was wanting. I tried to give her no more chances to let me down. I stopped waking her when I had a nightmare, sometimes after a lengthy internal debate. I refused to have babysitters, claiming that I was capable of taking care of myself. These actions made me proud and brought out the best in her; it was a mutually convincing facsimile of being grown up. My intention was to shield her from anxiety so completely that she could never again have an occasion to doubt herself; to accomplish this I became anxious for two. It ended up making me an unusually empathic therapist, but it swamped me with emotions I had no resources to metabolize. The purpose and the price went unnoticed until the day she died, when I no longer needed to pay it.

For the longest time I had an intimation that something in my past didn't compute. Was she as strong as she looked? If I was actually so secure, so adored (in between the bad episodes), why had anxiety that felt incapacitating plagued me my whole life? If she and I were so close, why did I feel so alone? Was I somehow to blame? How did I come to choose my vocation as a therapist at the age of ten (I have the letter I wrote her from camp to prove it)? These are the kinds of questions I've asked my patients for thirty-five years but never have adequately answered for myself before.

My mother stimulated me, encouraged me, and admired me, but she could never soothe me. Well before I had words to understand my experience, I never felt secure in her arms or confident that she could figure out how to make me comfortable without taking my discomfort as a sign of her inadequacy. The boundary, always too permeable between us, disintegrated under stress. Then I would become the mirror that reflected back not her best face but rather its unbearable underside—a dangerous thing for either one of us to see. So I learned to fit in, to feign comfort I didn't feel, not to need what she couldn't provide. The result was a silent despair that anyone would ever be attuned to me, and it had the effect of magnifying inborn sensitivities that neither one of us could handle. She recounted to me more than once, with ironic pride, that when I ran into something at age five and passed out in front of her, she fainted dead away and had to be revived herself. She took it as natural, even as a sign of laudable maternal instinct, that my anxiety made her intolerably anxious. I could only conclude there was no help for me.

My mother and I had an unspoken pact that met both our needs: I sustained her so subtly that she thought she was holding me. She couldn't tolerate and never admitted human weaknesses in herself, just like she never got sick; she didn't spend a day in bed all the time I lived at home. I couldn't turn to anyone else without betraying her and undermining her self-esteem; when I was a teenager she accused me, with real pain and bitterness, of preferring my friends to her.

I had to guarantee that she would never know what I was doing to prop her up, so I thought of the episodes when she revealed her most damaged self as lapses or aberrations, not as glimpses of underpinnings of her personality as integral as her sense of style. My way of protecting her from the devastating knowledge of her intermittent but profound failures was not to acknowledge them myself.

⁊∾⁊

My parents did eventually design and build their dream house in the suburbs and settled into the trappings of haute-bourgeois contentment. But a deep reservoir of suppressed malaise was already poisoning their genuine mutual affection.

I was fourteen when my mother first discovered signs that my father, unlikely as it seemed from his retiring demeanor, was an adulterer. He denied it, and she chose to believe him, or at least to suspend her disbelief. A year and a half later, when renewed suspicion prompted her to open his mail for the first time in her life, the evidence (bills for a car, furniture, and clothes she hadn't bought and a rent statement for an apartment at a hitherto unknown address) was inescapable. She showed up at my high school that afternoon with a suitcase full of my clothes and announced that we were moving out of our house and into a hotel.

But she could not stop there. She needed a witness, someone to validate her perception and vindicate her outrage, and it had to be me. Over my tears and frantic resistance, she insisted that I alone—not her sister who lived in the neighborhood, not a friend—accompany her to that apartment; of course she managed to get the keys from the super. There we had to go together from room to room, noting every detail of an environment (the robin's-egg-blue Princess phone stands out) entirely devoid of her trademark panache or palette. Afterward, when the only thing I wanted was to rush back home to my own room and bolt the door, she was furious with me. How could I want to desert her when I had a duty to perform?

But she could not stop there. When she moved us back home a week later—he promised to mend his ways—she demanded that the apartment be dismantled and that the ugly furniture, the carpet, and the car be handed over to me; for once she had no trouble giving a direct order, and he complied. She interpreted my angry tears—I hated everything but the car, and wanted no part of the spoils or my role as enforcer—as ingratitude. (A decade later, when she came to New York to help me move out of the apartment I shared with another secretive, unfaithful physician, she did give me a heartfelt apology, precious because it was so rare.)

Things never felt the same after we returned. The house had become a stage set, not a real place with a real family, and I fled, making more and more of myself off-limits and spending as much time as possible in what passed for bohemia in Cincinnati. She didn't let me go without a fight. I thought she was trying to control me, but now I know she was actually struggling frantically not to drown as her life preserver took on a life of its own and swam away.

It was then that I discovered music. Music had surrounded me my whole life—every member of my family played an instrument, and I spent hours singing folk songs and accompanying myself on the guitar, but this was another experience entirely. This was music not as a performance or a means of self-expression, but as a different kind of company than I had ever known. Decades before Walkmans and iPods, when stereo was young and tape recorders behemoths, Glenn Gould playing Bach on the piano became the companion of my solitude, transporting me to a world of order, clarity, and resolution, where passion and grief were expressed but manageable, life made sense, and consolation was possible. I didn't have to do anything or be anything to receive its balm. It has been my lullaby, my refuge in pain and fear, ever since. It took my mother's place, and it was so private she couldn't be jealous.

～○～

Even though both of us knew that I'd never be back, I didn't lose her entirely when I went away to college in Chicago. I visited, called, and wrote regularly—many of my letters were filled with a budding psychologist's good but unheeded advice on how to handle my brother's continuing difficulties—and received regular care packages of food and outfits; a spotted rabbit fur coat was included to keep me warm in the arctic winters. One night she showed up on the doorstep of my apartment unexpectedly after discovering evidence of yet another of my father's long-standing affairs, and I remember feeling hugely relieved that now she was on my turf and not the other way around. As expected, she returned home. When I went to New York City for graduate school, and for the rest of my life, she accepted the move with a characteristic mixture of fatalism, envy, and pride.

These dramatic gestures of flight, of which the Chicago trip was the last, must have given her the illusion of autonomy she never truly claimed. She stayed with my father as his health deteriorated, nursing him with a strange mixture of devotion and martyred obligation, moving once again into his hospital room, until he died when I was thirty-two. By then I was deeply estranged from him and felt numb at his funeral; I only reccovered our bond twenty years later when I wrote a book about him. I married two years later; not surprisingly she behaved outrageously at the wedding (catching my bouquet, offending my friends, and at one point making me cry because she felt she was being shunted aside forever) although she came to love my husband much less ambivalently than she could love me as an adult. When he became seriously ill, she could not do enough to help us both; her generosity in certain kinds of adversity always rang true.

She certainly seemed to prosper after my father's death. I think her self-esteem was no longer crushed by having tolerated humiliation for so long; she had endured. She looked and acted freer and seemed quite content to live alone now that she had to. Although she was astonishingly active mentally and physically—getting a job at the art museum shop, exercising, traveling, reading, going to parties and lunch, and finding a man who was enthralled with her—she never let herself get genuinely close to anybody again. She rarely had visitors in that ninety-foot-long house and inhabited increasingly less of it as time went by. It became her exoskeleton, her fortress against the perils of intimacy. Eventually she closed off the part that had been my father's office.

We were never again easy in each other's company. It grieved me, but I couldn't change it. Every visit, mine and hers, ended with her picking a fight; it was the only way she could separate. Shopping was the one bond that endured and satisfied, although by then I was selecting the clothes for her. Giving her presents was the one thing I could always do right because I understood her taste perfectly; I knew instinctively how to please her, in that arena at least, as long as she lived.

The exception to the now-chronic tension between us was her reaction when I published my first book at age forty-nine. I was girded for the worst. She could easily have found reason to take offense even though I dedicated it to her; it was, after all, about why I chose not to have children, and our relationship had figured prominently in that decision. But she surprised me. She was absolutely thrilled, and it really was for me, not about her own reflected glory. One of the best presents I ever gave her—as good as the wittiest outfit—was calling her from the green room at *The Today Show* and telling her to turn on her television and watch me. I didn't bask in the glow of her unalloyed joy like that again until I called her for the last time a decade later when she was on her deathbed.

But after that interlude, disappointment reasserted itself, as it had to, because my life was elsewhere. Over time it became less onerous to go to her fortress than to have her visit my apartment; in either place, though, I felt both compelled and unable to entertain her, and claustrophobia quickly set in. She was always glad to see me—I came armed with her favorite delicacies and my fetching husband—but her references to my imminent departure started soon and quickly drained her pleasure away. Abandonment seemed to be the only thing that was real for her. Even when she had her own life at last, she behaved as if she had nothing, and was nothing, without me. I always marveled that some of my friends actually looked forward to spending time with their mothers and wished they lived closer. My own visits got ever shorter, the intervals between them longer.

Telephone conversations were no easier. Her answers to my comments or questions—she rarely initiated anything—were increasingly monosyllabic and always delivered with an accusatory undertone. Why couldn't she ever just say that she missed me, that she wanted to see me, or ask about what I was doing and really want to know? I hated to see that the person who had hung so avidly on every detail of my activities, whom I had to flee to avoid being engulfed, was shutting me out in a distorted notion of self-defense. Although I am rarely at a loss for words, I struggled to find anything to say to fill the growing void between us. I was hungry for contact, repairing, remembering; we used to be able to do it. Our time was fleeing fast; I didn't want it filled with talk about the weather.

Then she started getting lost while driving, for hours at a time. Since she seemed to take it in stride and I had inherited her hopeless sense of direction, I thought nothing of it but pressed her to investigate because she was eighty-seven. Her doctor, whom she had ensorcelled long ago, had no idea that anything was wrong. Neither he nor I could believe the diagnosis of incipient dementia.

The news flattened me. Far worse than anticipating the logistics of arranging for her care from six hundred miles away, worse even than contemplating the horror of such a fate for someone whose mind and memory and late-won freedom meant everything to her, was the certain knowledge that now I could never get her back.

Some of what I miserably foresaw came true. Her personality, though still unmistakable, was increasingly hollowed out, and our already difficult times together became excruciating exercises in obligation and regret. At the same time, I felt an urgency about telling her that I loved her and was proud of her while she could still comprehend; despite all my other feelings, it was true. Sadly, she always seemed surprised to hear it, as though in unguarded moments she didn't feel that she deserved it. It tormented me that the early ravages of her fiendish illness, coupled with her increasingly vain attempts to maintain appearances, made genuine contact impossible. I was struck by the irony that now, when I really wanted to, I could do nothing to comfort her. So I tried to mourn in anticipation and salvage what I could before I lost even the shell.

Then I had the miraculous luck to find Linda, the geriatric case manager who became my surrogate sister, my "couples' therapist," and my friend. She and the staff she assembled to care for my mother after we had to move her to an assisted living apartment at age eighty-nine—four tenderhearted women and one adoring ex-marine—eased my burden and gave her the kind of attention she had always craved. They also gave me six new pairs of eyes.

I had never watched anybody else interact with my mother in my role before, and it was riveting. Even with only part of her brain operative, she ferreted out each aide's hidden talents and managed to make herself indispensable. She encouraged her favorite, in whom she discerned artistic ability, to pursue photography (it was she who took the reclining portrait that captured my mother so perfectly). The dowdy one's wardrobe and makeup got a makeover, the self-effacing one got informal assertiveness training, and the depressed ex-marine, naturally, got a nonagenarian girlfriend. A letter I found from the lively young animal lover who had moved out of town contained paint chips and requested decorating advice. "Dear Esther," it read, "I remember you had a blouse that you loved because it was the color of the sky, so I thought I'd like a room to look like that. What shade would you recommend?" She also regularly "fired" every one of them for infractions I was all too familiar with—being late, or getting sick, or getting married, or otherwise demonstrating that they had lives of their own. The crime of reminding her that she was dependent was still punishable by exile. However, since she wasn't paying their salaries and had a much shorter memory than she used to, they had the luxury of being able to ignore her.

It was painful to see these loving strangers enjoy her and navigate her demands when I could not. But, I reasoned, they were not her children and so had a built-in buffer that I lacked. I also was able to appreciate what I had gotten by seeing her lavish it on them. In accepting that I, too, was relying on them, I stopped feeling guilty that the best I could do was arrange what she gratefully called "this service," and that it was more effective than I could ever be. A way had presented itself for me to provide for her at one remove.

Most important were Linda's insights. She told me what she saw, explained things I was too close or too hurt to understand. She repeated anything positive my mother said about me in my absence or that she intuited that my mother felt but could not express—and suppressed the rest. This tiny, indomitable woman was fiercely protective but clearheaded about both my mother's magical and her hateful sides, and squarely faced the desperate neediness and terror under the crumbling façade. It was she who made possible my mother's extraordinary death and arranged what I never imagined I would have—the shining best of her at the eleventh hour.

A heart attack at ninety put an end to her exercising and eventually to walking at all, but the only thing she complained about—though far less than before—was my absence. She stopped calling me, probably because she couldn't remember the number, but she kept sending checks for my husband's and my birthdays and for our anniversary as long as she could write. She fought the indignities of age and infirmity with every ounce of her formidable will.

On three occasions we rushed back to Cincinnati because it looked like she was dying. The last of these false alarms came just after I had arrived at my country house one summer morning. Considering how estranged we were, I was taken aback by how frantic I felt to get back in time to say good-bye. Before we sped to the airport, I ran to my garden and picked her the most fragrant, startling, voluptuous bouquet of flowers and leaves and grasses I could collect. As we waited to board amid escalating flight delays, I ran around the terminal madly trying to find an outlet to charge my phone so at least I could hear her voice one last time and tell her what she meant to me. When we finally arrived that evening, she was sitting up in bed. She casually greeted us, admired the flowers, and said offhandedly that she was glad we'd stopped by. This rehearsal told me I was far more involved with her than I had any idea.

The last time I saw her was her ninety-second birthday. She was holding court at the head of the table in her favorite restaurant, dressed to the nines. Even in her wheelchair, she looked every inch a self-possessed if slightly vacant queen surveying her courtiers, wearing without irony the gold paper crown one of them had bought for her and insisting that everybody eat the foods she liked best and drink champagne to her health. The next month, with Linda's masterful and discreet assistance, she gave an engagement party for one of her caretakers—the one she finally forgave for getting married. She wanted every ounce of living and savored every moment in the world. Overriding doctors' orders, she flatly refused any treatment that would interfere with her enjoying life, even though it might prolong it. Until her last week, she insisted on being taken out to lunch whenever she was strong enough to sit up. I was struck that the woman who had been so terrified to live alone when she was young and healthy that she stayed in a marriage that demeaned her, showed not the slightest fear of dying forty years later.

Then, suddenly, the end really was nigh. It was early December, and I had just gotten back from a vacation in South America when Linda called to tell me that my mother had been given a day at most to live. "I know it's real this time, Jeanne," she said decisively. "She's said good-bye to her cat."

"Shall I leave right now?" I asked.

"You really don't have to come. She doesn't want you to see her like this—she doesn't want to worry you," she told me with the combination of directness and unfailing compassion that characterized every conversation we'd had for five years. This time I was absolutely furious.

"Worry me!" I spit out. "She's not thinking about me at all, any more than when she dragged me to that goddamn apartment. She's abandoning me and pretending to take care of me, like always. She won't let me comfort her—she can't even let me say good-bye. The goddamn cat means more to her than I do."

My husband joined the chorus of "she's trying to protect you in her way," but I was having none of it. I didn't believe it; so many things that were supposedly for my sake had really been for hers. Was narcissism masquerading as selflessness all there was in the end?

I struggled to accept that our final exchange would have to be long-distance. What could I possibly say to her? This really was my last chance. I didn't want to be cold, or just go through the motions. I wanted to be real, and I wanted to be an adult. I tried to put my rage aside; I knew there was grief underneath.

Linda told me to call around noon, when she thought my mother would be strong enough to speak to me. She told me that, despite labored breathing and flickering consciousness, my mother was marshaling all her resources for the occasion. I forced myself to focus and think straight. I had two hours.

Then, unbidden, an image of my mother as a young woman with her own mother—an old family snapshot I'd seen many times—came to mind. In it, my grandmother was younger than when I knew her, but just as clueless, just as frightened of life, staring blankly in front of her and barely inhabiting her body. Now, though, I literally saw my mother being the adult for both of them, her vitality and air of authority masking—even then—her fear of failing at the Sisyphean task of caretaking. Standing slightly in the background, she was steadying her mother's arm and holding her mother's purse as well as her own, with a naturalness that indicated this happened all the time. I realized I had never before seen any other woman give her purse to another woman to hold if she could help it. Suddenly it was clear to me that my mother must have vowed, whether she knew it or not, to spare me her fate. She would never "worry" me by exposing me to any behavior that (by her idiosyncratic standard) smacked of weakness, neediness, or incompetence. Unlike her own mother, she would always take care of me as she defined it, letting me be the child she should have been in the way she should have been—whether it was what I needed or not. To her dying day, she would be a better mother than the one she had, never leaning on me—always carrying her own purse. Although there were times when I had to carry her as she clung to it, the intention was honorable, if misguided. I felt a flood of gratitude that I had figured this out in time to tell her.

Giving her ample opportunity to symbolically put on her makeup, and summoning all the resolve and calm in a crisis I'd learned from her, I dialed.

"Hello, darling!" she said with complete self-possession and lucidity. "You're just back from Buenos Aires, aren't you? Did you have a good time?"

I had called her on my return just three days before, when she didn't remember that I'd gone. "Mother," I said, cutting to the chase, "this may be our last conversation, and there's something I want to tell you."

"What are you talking about? I'm fine," she demurred with hearty, almost credible, conviction.

Pressing on, I said, "I want you to know that I know how important it was for you to take care of me, and you did it."

She dropped the façade, the infomercial of business as usual, hoping that she'd heard what she thought she'd heard, and said with astonishment, "Really? I did? You *know* that?"

"Yes, you did. You took care of me," I said with a tenderness that I hadn't been able to muster for decades, that for the first time cost me nothing because it was the truth.

"Thank you!" she whispered joyously, almost rapturously—words my mother had rarely uttered, and in a tone she had never used, in the fifty-seven-and-a-half years of our acquaintance. I knew she was thanking me for everything. The last words we spoke to each other were our first of mutual acknowledgment and consolation.

❧

The next day she died in her own bed, under that tiger-striped throw, as she wished. Her favorite caregiver, who stayed by her side the whole time, told me what happened. In her last hour, she regained consciousness long enough to exclaim, with quiet fervor, "What a beautiful moment in time. Very few people ever see this. This is my day." Although I wasn't there, nobody had to explain what she meant. This was no simple statement of fact; it was her hard-won credo, her affirmation: "Even the day I die, my last day on earth, belongs to me. This is *my* day. I rejoice in it."

Death had no dominion over her love of life, and in the end she prevailed.

❧

I didn't cry as much at her funeral as Linda and the staff did, all wearing gifts she had given them. The young woman who was an animal lover pointed out the flock of birds circling overhead, as if to see her off. How poignant it was, I thought, that a human being so much larger than life could have ashes light and insubstantial enough to fit in a cigar box with room to spare.

After the party in her honor that she had ordained, I stopped at her apartment on my way to the airport, and gathered up some more photographs, the red suede mary janes I had given her, her fish necklace, and copies of my books. In the jumble of thrift-shop finds filling one of her drawers, I discovered a pair of over-size red-rimmed sunglasses with loose eyepieces that I had never seen before, and I snatched them up. The first thing I did when I got home was to have the lenses replaced with dark grey ones of my own: the beginning, I knew, of a different way of seeing.

The Birth of Hope

Back in New York that night I found myself wandering around my apartment, gazing hungrily at the things that reminded me of her—the Navajo rugs, the old hat mold she used to display as a sculpture, the quirky prints and African hangings—the atmosphere I had created, a combination of our sensibilities, that owed so much to her. They made me feel a little less bereft because they were imbued with her spirit. Though I felt surrounded by her presence in their presence, the universe seemed diminished without her. I was surprised that I felt bereft at all; as expected, mostly I felt relieved for both of us that her death had been so meaningful and that we had had the extraordinary good fortune to find each other at the end. The weight that had descended precipitously upon me as soon as she was diagnosed began imperceptibly to lift now that my job was done.

But I didn't miss her. As much as I missed her being in the world, I felt no longing to interact with her. Appreciating and admiring her did not cancel out how difficult it had been to be her daughter, especially for the last quarter century when so little felt real.

This admission began my inquiry into my mother's character—now that I had placed, literally as well as symbolically, my "lenses" in her "glasses"—to try to make sense of the welter of contradictory emotions she inspired in me. I felt the full force of how difficult it is to see one's mother accurately. How ultimately mysterious any mother is; you think you should know each other best, that you have a certain private, almost involuntary knowledge because you once shared a body, but in fact you're far too close, too full of needs and projections to grasp her essence as a stranger or a peer might. Rarely do you get even a momentary glimpse, as I was granted at the end, of her hidden truth.

Death makes all the difference; it broadens your perspective. I had tried to see her before, but until then the effort of simply coping with her and the feelings she evoked got in the way. You have a three-dimensional view when you're no longer face-to-face; you can see inside and around the back. Suddenly I could imagine what my mother was like before I ever met her—when she was a daughter, a sister, a wife, my brother's mother, when neither of us had yet been fixed in each other's sights. Now I could also see us together from a therapeutic distance—beyond blame, beyond the frantic need to get through or justify myself, beyond disappointment, beyond rage—beyond fear. Being freed from the grip of not daring to know gave me the courage to proceed.

I started by taking my reactions, especially the uncomfortable ones, seriously and considering their implications no matter where they led; they were my source of information about some secret between us that I had to decipher. Like a detective, I decided to examine every assumption, follow every lead; my quarry was my own previously inexplicable and unfixable anxiety and despair. The determination that was my proudest inheritance came to my aid.

The first thing I noticed was how I behaved right after she died, how I had instinctively connected with her through the objects and décor in my apartment. When I feared that I had lost or damaged anything special of hers I felt miserable, as though I were losing a living part of her. Why did I do that rather than replay tender scenes, memories, wordless moments of intimacy? I admired and loved her most for her potent personal qualities and their manifestations, not the way I felt when we were together. The full force of my unavoidable conclusion hit me: something fundamentally maternal had always been missing. She wasn't primarily cold or distant, but I never could turn to her when I was scared. Because of her I could swim, I could cook, I could decorate and write and live with intensity, but—despite her sincere best efforts—I could never feel all right just because she was there.

A dream confirmed this painful recognition. In it, I bumped into an acquaintance of mine, someone whose mother had recently died. "Joe," I said. "I've just been thinking about you. I was so moved by your dream." Then I began to weep and was still sobbing when I awoke. The dream within my dream, which Joe had actually recounted to me in waking life, was about weeping like an infant himself, and then feeling blissful comfort when he was uplifted in his mother's loving arms, an experience that rekindled his childhood trust in God. I wept because now I knew that no arms ever lifted me like that, so there was no fundamental trust to rekindle. I had to find out why.

ᥱᦞᥱ

Now I had the fundamental information I needed to address this question. My next step was to take inventory of my mother's personality just as I had of her possessions, deciding what to keep, what to discard, and how to integrate those selections into my own, now separate, mental household. Of course, she had wanted me to take everything. I understood that this process was far from entirely in my conscious control—otherwise why would we all be stuck with so many of our parents' traits that we would do anything to get rid of?—but I thought the effort would add focus to an undertaking that was rarely conducted rationally. I hoped to cultivate receptivity, just as I'd done by looking at photographs of her. I hadn't been able to attempt anything like this when my father had died twenty-five years ago; I didn't want to miss my only other opportunity.

I divided my legacy from her into four categories: the first two—what I got from her that I treasured, and what I didn't get that I regretted missing—were fairly straightforward. The third—what I

got that I wanted to get rid of—took work to confront, but was
no mystery. The fourth category—what I needed and didn't get
because she didn't have it—was unknown territory, inconceivable
until now.

My Psychological Inventory

1. WHAT I GOT THAT I TREASURED

I marveled at the guts and gallantry with which my mother maintained her identity despite onslaughts that would have shattered
most people. Her joie de vivre was as unstoppable as her ability to
encourage and appreciate those she cared about. She gave me determination so powerful that I feel confident it will never desert
me, either. A dream, my usual source of inner information, confirmed my conclusion: The teacher of an onerous, frustrating, ex-
hausting class, in which I was one of the very few participants
who stayed until the end, asked me what I had gotten out of it.
"Only one thing—endurance," I answered, "but it was worth it."

2. WHAT I DIDN'T GET THAT I REGRETTED MISSING

My mother had a natural social ease all her life that I did not inherit, any more than her ability to play the piano by ear. With it
came unshakable confidence in her own appeal; I never quite trust
my own. These deficits, along with not getting those legs, I have
come to accept.

3. WHAT I GOT THAT I WANTED TO GET RID OF

Then I tackled the harder questions, the ones that forced me to
take an inventory of my own least appealing attributes. What
qualities and habits of mind that were originally hers did I long to
expunge? The most toxic ones on the list were insidious; these

were things she expressed not so much by what she said as by how she behaved, often unwittingly. I had absorbed them just as involuntarily and would have to exert all my inherited will to exorcise or disarm them.

Because it was the bane of our relationship, I took special note of how she had reacted to my visits, when only my eventual departure was real. From this (and it was only the most recent example) I realized I had deduced that the negative always trumps the positive because its value is so much stronger—a conviction that causes you to undervalue anything good until, over time, it hardly registers. Then you cannot feel it has staying power, and you cannot be sustained by good memories. Abandonment was my mother's bottom line; she spent her life trying magically to protect herself against it by catastrophic expectation. It's hard to reconcile such profound pessimism with her exuberance and resilience, but people are full of contradictions. She had a lifelong lack of basic trust, which she unintentionally bequeathed to me. I don't want to keep it.

My mother also confused disappointment—which for her included disagreement—with desertion; in her assessment of people's characters, too, the bad outweighed the good. With the exception of my father, she wrote them off for the slightest infraction and slammed the door on those—virtually everyone she knew—who failed even momentarily to support her. Her threshold for disillusionment was extremely low; there was no room for second chances, for working things out, for trying to see from someone else's point of view. If you got back in her good graces, it was because she was bestowing, like God, undeserved forgiveness for your trespasses. I fight my own tendency to do the same by reminding myself repeatedly what really matters in the people I love—and by remembering with gratitude that they do the same for me. Of course, to do this you have to be aware of your own shortcomings, an ability my mother lacked; enumerating my own was an important way to differentiate myself from her.

Perfectionism cut off so many opportunities for my mother. It was her tormenting, hidden self-doubt, I am convinced, that caused her to judge others so harshly; in fact, she set a far more draconian standard for herself. Since everything had always depended on her, she dared not falter. In her system there was no place for problems, or for learning from experience; when nobody backs you up, everything has to be right the first time. She blinded herself to her own mother's ineptness by rushing in to fill the gap. I realized with a jolt that I was perpetuating that very pattern, although the gap I had to fill was not an abyss, as hers had been.

4. WHAT I NEEDED THAT SHE WASN'T ABLE TO GIVE

One of the reasons she couldn't learn to be a good enough mother—one who could function when her children got anxious— was that she couldn't tolerate her perfectly normal failure to be one effortlessly from the start. She had no mother to emulate in this regard, so she panicked at the first sign of trouble. This ultimately left her hopeless and alone, convinced that she was an unlovable failure, until illness left her no choice but to relax her standards. Then she became more tolerant and happier; she had the mother(s) she needed at last.

I began to listen anew to that unmistakable Voice of Authority, and heard nuances I'd never noticed before. It conveyed much more than aesthetic or moral judgments; she used it to reaffirm her supreme competence, which was always in doubt, with such conviction that I believed her as long as she lived. Only when The Voice was silenced did it become less awe-inspiring.

Some of her pronouncements were truly smart and wise, but many had an authoritarian edge, a rigidity masked as certainty—

always the sign of insecurity underneath. Proclaiming "Red is a neutral" as a philosophy of life is extravagant and original, but there's no room for nuance; in certain circumstances it can be monotonous or just plain wrong. Red is vivid and alive—the color of life—but it neutralizes everything around it.

Until I replaced her lenses with my own, I saw the world through my mother's glasses. I never questioned her premises; I never thought of them as premises at all. Doing so is the final separation, made possible by her death alone. To celebrate my independence I created my own list of principles to live by:

Esther's Laws of Nature—Revised

1. Life is not predictably doom-filled. It is doom- and delight-filled.
2. Leave room to be wrong occasionally. It actually feels good.
3. People do not always disappoint in the end, and sometimes even disappointing ones come through. Accept flawed love.
4. Betrayal doesn't offend your pride, it destroys your soul. Don't rationalize it; don't tolerate it.
5. Red is a very noisy neutral, and it doesn't always play well with other colors. Just because you could use it with everything doesn't mean you should.

❦

Strengthened and encouraged by my efforts so far—and pleased that I could still laugh and think of her fondly—I was ready to confront the hardest, deepest wound of all: the nadir I hit when I can't see my way out of illness or some other threatening situation, the dread I have no words to express because it is so primordial.

The essential step was realizing there was something to investigate. A question occurred to me that I had never asked myself before: why did I assume that I was doomed to be stuck with unmodifiable terror forever, that my reactions could not change and I would never feel better? My impotence was simply a given, written in stone, not a conviction that I had reasons for feeling or that might be transformed if I understood its origin or its function in my life. I assumed this despairing state of mind and body was static, not dynamic—simply the awful truth about me.

I don't think that way about anything, or anybody, else. I passionately believe, and tell my patients, that the only power that can never be taken away is your ability to change your relationship to thoughts and feelings—that the act of observing changes nature. There must be some powerful reason why I considered the most disturbing of my own reactions "objective" fact, exempt from my own fundamental belief. This perverse and frightening version of the unquestionable Voice of Authority had all the hallmarks of the way my mother operated; she had to be implicated.

When I looked for an explanation, I discovered why I assumed that nobody could console me. It was my way to preserve my mother as the center of my universe. She wanted desperately to provide basic security, but she couldn't do it because she'd never had it; I doubt that her own mother had ever had it, either. Since she also couldn't stand to know any of this, she blamed me for her failure. Her judgment had to be right, so I took the rap. Even though my father provided a calming antidote with his medical expertise, I had signed an exclusive contract that made her the sole source of all comfort, and I honored it even though she could not. Others gave up on their parents or saw their flaws earlier and stopped idealizing them, but I kept looking at her and to her for much longer than I should have, unable to seek what I needed elsewhere, thinking her deficit was mine.

The conclusion I reached was disturbing but ultimately liberating: there really was nothing inconsolable about me—I was just a sensitive kid who needed my mother to figure out how to soothe me. I had spent my whole life thinking I was beyond help because the alternative was worse; I had given up on myself rather than give up on her.

～～

Finally I knew what to do; I had to look for help in all the right places. I found it all around me, including where I least expected it. I also found it inside me. When I didn't have to be so perfect, when my shortcomings in the self-consolation department didn't seem so fixed or fatal, I discovered that I had more resources than I ever imagined. What I needed was hiding in plain sight.

The swimming pool, my mother's element, has turned out to be my training ground for fear management, with a woman young enough to be my own daughter as my guide.

I had swum for years, but soon after my mother died—undoubtedly as a way to connect with her—I decided to go to swim school. The ease and fluency of moving beautifully in the water appealed as I approached sixty, and I wanted to learn the butterfly and improve my freestyle. I found an innovative program called Total Immersion ("Discover Your Inner Fish" is its motto) and began working with Cari, the nose-ringed daughter of the inventor of this new technique. My natural ability and well-honed skills as teacher's pet served me well, until I reached a gigantic obstacle: breathing to both sides. Not being able to get enough air as I struggled to learn the difficult coordination (the left side of my body has always felt as though it belonged to somebody else) induced the familiar feelings of panic and despair, both physical and psychological. Automatically I assumed I'd never learn, and that my teacher, sweet and sincere though she seemed, would give up on me. With my usual persistence, I practiced constantly, grimly determined—"muscling through" as one of my patients calls it—sometimes even coming close to crying in the water.

But then I tried something I'd never tried before. I told Cari I was scared and that I felt embarrassed to be having such a hard time. "Everybody's scared," she said, to my astonishment. Then she earnestly figured out what to do about it, telling me what had worked for her, standing next to me as I did every stroke. She suggested relaxing my face, and then breathing out slowly, to induce ease until I felt it. Then she taught me how to lie on my side, arm outstretched, to catch my breath between tries. "This is your wall when you have no wall," she explained. I started practicing differently, using my self-constructed wall—and imagining her beside me even in deep water, encouraging and instructing me. In a few months the skill was mine. I smiled as I swam, as though I'd been a fish forever.

My success inspired me to take another leap of faith; I decided I wanted a swimming pool of my own, one with a current, just big enough for me, to celebrate my birthday. We would have to build an addition to our house in upstate New York to put it in. We had the money to do it, but it was still an extravagance. As soon as my husband agreed, I panicked. Out of the blue, I thought (channeling another swimmer in my family), "What if I suddenly get sick, what if I die, and never get to use it? It's just something I'll have to risk," I told myself. "Life is uncertain, but it must be lived, or you die before you're dead." This is my day.

I added three more principles to my list of Esther's Laws:

6. Consolation and comfort often come from unlikely sources. Seek them out, and rejoice when you find them.
7. Usually when you get sick, you eventually get better. Even if you don't at the end, statistics are still in your favor until then.
8. Your own strength will surprise you even when you think it's gone.

༺❦༻

Something is happening. It's not noticeable to anybody but me yet, but I think I feel—dare I say it?—a little more hopeful. Hope does not mean the absence of despair, or the unshakable security someone with a different mother and a different past might know. I don't expect that, and I don't need it; my pessimistic core is part of me forever. But help does not feel entirely out of reach anymore.

The acid test happened just as I began to write about the meaning of my mother's death. It was a struggle to figure out, and to articulate all my feelings about her, because I had to reexperience everything I was trying to describe, and I wanted to do her justice. After a week of worrying that I would never be able to manage it, that even though I've written three autobiographies before I'd lost the knack, I found my way in and hit my stride—when a computer glitch wiped out everything I'd written. I fell into a pit of frantic misery that felt as bottomless as it ever had.

"I've learned nothing," I moaned. "I'll never get it back." As I paced from room to room, aimless and desperate, I decided to take a nap to gather myself together, and I had a dream.

The dream consisted of only one image: my scruffy but indestructible orange duffel bag of ballistic nylon, the one I take to the country every weekend, and that I joke is so cavernous that I could live inside. I unzipped it and found, to my surprise, that it contained two other bags that had come with it but that I'd never seen before, fully packed with everything I needed. This was a very different bag than the one my mother brought to my high school so many years ago.

The meaning was clear and instantly consoling: even when I felt bereft, I had a surfeit of inner resources. Some belonged to me, some had been given to me by other people who knew what I needed, but they sufficed. Since they were in my traveling bag, they were portable. I could take them anywhere, for the rest of my life.

I sat down again to write, calm and confident that I would recover everything that I had lost, and more besides.

～✦～

As I stood up at the end of my exercise session today, something unexpected happened. My trainer had put a two-and-a-half-pound weight on my head, as she often does, to help me find my natural balance. It's harder than it looks and always feels shaky and slightly scary at first, as though the disc could fall off and land on my foot. At that moment, I had a visual and sensory experience that startled me: I felt that I was surrounded by cushions of living light, soft and resilient. They were all around me. They kept me in place without any effort; I only had to give in and let myself be held by them. There was my father, and my friends, and my husband, and under it all was my mother, flawed but real. At last, I knew I was supported, physically supported, by love.

I teetered slightly as I tried to find true equilibrium, seeking a sense of standing erect but at ease, without locking and straining, trusting and feeling suspended in their midst. Their distilled love was all around me, palpable like flesh, keeping me upright, even though I wavered. Whether I could stay standing was no longer a question. My mother gave me what she could to get me started, and I got the rest for myself. There was no unfillable deficit anymore. I had enough; I never had to steel myself again. Her arms had not been able to hold me steady because none ever held her, but she hadn't dropped me, either. I stood on my own but not alone at last, sure and solid and supple, held yet free, energetic and still and secure, always accompanied. I stood, no longer a baby with no resources of her own, but upright, as an adult. It was active, it was conscious, and I was communicating with everyone who held me. Nothing could take them from me; they were part of me. I didn't have to force it or fear they would desert me in my hour of need ever again; the work was done, it was mine. I would not fall.

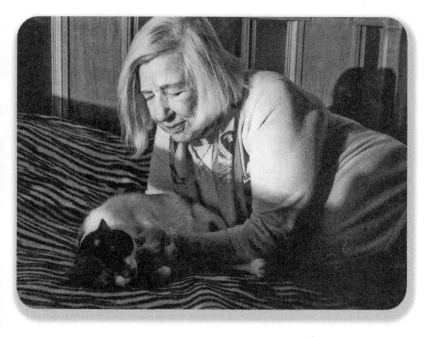

Esther at ninety

CHAPTER 2

Death Benefits

The Last Taboo

❧

A New Look at Loss

Parents die much later in their children's lives than ever before, so most adults now have the opportunity to discover and to cultivate death benefits, as I had the good fortune to do—if only they know where to look and how to go about it.

Just a few decades ago it was unusual for a midlife adult to have a living parent, but now an overlap of fifty years or more is common. In the twenty-first century, people tend to be thirty-five to fifty-four years old when their fathers die and between forty-five and sixty-four when their mothers die. Fifty percent of the population has lost both parents by age fifty-four, and 75 percent are orphans by age sixty-two; parents die as we age. This time frame is in itself an advantage not only because the relationship lasts so long—far longer than most marriages—but also because the large overlap means that by the time we lose them we have become adults and often parents ourselves; finally, we can empathize.

Curiously, the increased longevity of the parent/child relationship has not been accompanied by an increase in research about what happens when it ends. Though by far the most common type of bereavement, parent loss in adulthood is the least studied; the deaths of spouses, of young children's parents—even of older parents' adult children—get much more coverage. Sigmund Freud himself, who called the world's attention to hidden aspects of family dynamics, wrote astonishingly little about the subject; his most important contribution was the brief essay "Mourning and Melancholia," written early in his career and never expanded. There is virtually nothing else on the topic before 1980, and only three scientific papers on midlife women's loss of their mothers had been published as of 2002. Aside from self-help books aimed at bereaved baby boomers, the neglect continues.

Why has a phenomenon that profoundly alters the lives of 11.6 million adults every year—5 percent of the population of the United States—generated so little interest? The assumption that midlife loss of a parent is so common, so much "in the natural order of things" that it is uneventful, is widespread. Why bother studying something so obvious? Such literal-mindedness rationalizes and fuels avoidance. Anxiety over our own mortality is the real reason nobody looks too closely at the demise of the older generation; if we did, we would have to face that we are next in line. And though Freud wrote little about death and grief, he endured quite a lot of both in his life, beginning with the death of his young brother. The terror the topic generated was too much even for the man who fearlessly explored sex and aggression.

Since parental death is considered so normal and predictable, people are shocked and unprepared for the intensity of their reactions when it happens. Few adults expect to feel unmoored, depressed, shaken, or numbed—let alone relieved—by the loss of parents who may seem peripheral to their current lives. As a result, they have to negotiate this major psychological transition without knowledge or guidance.

Defining orphanhood as a nonevent robs it of transformative power. Many fail to recognize its impact or to relate parent loss to significant changes in their lives. A fifty-year-old advertising executive told me that her mother's recent death at age eighty-nine was upsetting "even though" she was aged. In the course of our conversation, she mentioned offhandedly that for the first time in her life she had recently found herself buying clothes. This woman, who had never had much interest in fashion and who had a decided resistance to spending money on herself, had suddenly acquired a stylish and costly new wardrobe. When I asked whether her expenditures had any relationship to her loss, she was astonished that she hadn't made the connection; her mother had not bought a new outfit in years. Although her mother's self-denial had always troubled her daughter, she had unconsciously emulated it until her gleeful posthumous shopping spree. Without knowing why, she was dressing herself for success in the next phase of her own life.

Guilt is the other reason midlife parent loss is ignored—guilt about being released from emotional demands or caretaking burdens ("It's such a comfort to know that the phone's not going to ring in the middle of the night," a dutiful son admitted to me), guilt about profiting financially, and—most deeply buried of all—guilt about surviving. Unconsciously, every human being is relieved when death happens to somebody else, even to a beloved parent. Ambivalence is integral to all intimate relationships; those we love and need have power over us. Since parents are the most central of all, part of us secretly wants them dead so that we can be free. This wish is even more powerful, and less acceptable, when the relationship is conflicted.

The very things that make parents irreplaceable allow us to come fully into our own only when they depart. Our relationship with them is the template for all others, including our relationship with ourselves; the physical resemblance reinforces the psychic one. I recall taking a dance class with my mother when I was in my forties. A friend of hers was standing between us at the ballet bar, and when we turned to do a step on the other side, she started laughing; "I feel like I'm in a hall of mirrors," she said. Unbeknownst to either my mother or me, our movements replicated each other's. When asked to visualize a man or a woman, sixty- and seventy-year-olds still describe their parents; the first faces we see are our touchstones forever.

Our role in the world changes when there is no longer anybody to answer to, to turn to, or to rebel against. We become the final authority, the "adult"; the buck stops with us. Whether we were estranged or inseparable from our parents (or a combination of both) in their lifetimes, their deaths leave us truly alone—and truly in charge—for the first time.

Parent loss gets much less attention than it deserves, but the positive effects of parent loss get practically none at all. Personal distress accounts for some of the blindness of researchers who are themselves anticipating or experiencing the very losses they would be investigating. Death benefits also take time— sometimes decades—to unfold, and most studies of bereavement examine only the acute phase of mourning, when negative reactions usually predominate. Shame is another major impediment. To profit psychologically from a parent's demise seems to negate love and loyalty; admitting personal gains is suspect, and enjoying them is taboo. "It would be like dancing on my mother's grave," a patient of mine explained.

The most insidious enemy of death benefits is the pervasive assumption that personality is fixed by midlife and that major inner or outer change is by then a thing of the past. Who can appreciate, much less cultivate, something that has been defined out of existence?

Despite all the prohibitions, midlife is an ideal time to profit from the potent experience of losing a parent. At last we are equipped to have some perspective on the past and to take responsible chances on the future. Self-reliance becomes more appealing, and less dangerous, when you already have a well-established personal and professional identity; it is no accident that entrepreneurs over forty have the most successful start-up businesses. Since death is the ultimate separation, when it happens you no longer have to work to create distance from a deceased parent or feel guilty about needing to do so; there is no parental home not to visit anymore. And the dead cannot be offended when their offspring oppose them, disappoint them, or fail to consult them. Their notions of propriety in sex, religion, or lifestyle need not be yours ever again. Even the happiest childhood has aspects worth leaving behind.

Freud never analyzed death benefits, but he did experience them—as did Anna Freud, his daughter and heir. The founder of psychoanalysis was forty years old when his eighty-one-year-old father died, and seventy-four (and suffering from cancer himself) when his mother died at the age of ninety-five. Both deaths had a revolutionary impact on his work, but he and his biographers only recognized the significance of his father's. Freud wrote that he felt "uprooted" by his father's death and mourned him intensely, although their relationship had been conflicted. Soon afterward, he wrote *The Interpretation of Dreams*, his most important work, and formulated the Oedipus complex (named for the Greek myth in which Oedipus unwittingly kills his father and marries his mother), which was to become the cornerstone of his mature theory. The centrality of a son's competition with his father for his mother's love became clear to him only after he himself had won it by outliving his rival.

Freud's reaction to his mother's death was strange indeed. Although he adored her, he reported feeling no grief (because she was old and ill, he claimed); he did not attend her funeral (he sent Anna), ostensibly because of his own illness—excuses he would easily have seen through if a patient had made them, but which have, astonishingly, been accepted at face value until recently. Four months afterward he wrote his first paper devoted explicitly to the topic of female sexuality and also explored the earliest phase of development in which the mother is omnipotent—and which he labeled the "pre-Oedipal" phase—for the first time. He wrote to his closest friend that his mother's death caused an "increase in personal freedom" and predicted that "the value of life will somehow have changed noticeably in the deeper layers." Only then, so near death himself, could he separate enough from his intense relationship with her to begin to understand it; to think of women as powerful and sexual beings was far too threatening while she was alive.

Freud's death had a similarly beneficial effect on his youngest daughter, Anna. The only one of Freud's children to follow his profession (and to be her father's patient), Anna worshipped him and served as his caretaker as well as the guardian of his intellectual legacy at the end of his life. After his death, she overcame her shyness and fear of travel to become the leader of the psychoanalytic movement and took the field in new directions in her writing. She found her own voice only after he died, demonstrating that death benefits can occur even when the most intimate of bonds is severed.

Although psychologists have failed to recognize death benefits, novelists have not. Princess Maria, Prince Andrey's self-effacing sister in Leo Tolstoy's *War and Peace*, begins to feel them immediately after her admirable but tyrannical father dies:

> Unconsciously she sat up, smoothed her hair, got to her feet and walked over to the window, instinctively drawing into her lungs the freshness of the clear but windy evening.
>
> "Yes, now you can enjoy your fill of the evening! He is gone, and there is no one to hinder you," she said to herself.

From then on, this dutiful daughter becomes more womanly as well as more forceful and eventually marries.

Recent research has validated what Tolstoy understood and Freud and his daughter lived out—that the death of a parent makes a significant difference for adults, most often for the better. Every one of the rare investigations that has looked for such benefits has found them, and in a majority of cases. In one study, sixty-nine percent of survivors felt as though they were different people after their parents died, with "fewer obstacles to life." Subjects in another study enjoyed improved physical health in the five years after bereavement; they were determined to take better care of themselves than their parents had done.

Two-thirds also made changes in their careers or private lives that they attributed to improved self-esteem and newfound freedom; they felt liberated by no longer having to please their parents or worry about the consequences of their displeasure. Even the suffering and stress of mourning does not prevent growth; subjects who were anxious and depressed still made positive changes in their lives.

One of the most provocative pieces of evidence for death benefits has been hiding in a psychiatric journal since 1950. Not surprisingly, the finding has never been followed up. Two psychiatrists at a large metropolitan mental hospital discovered, to their amazement, that three young acute paranoid schizophrenics, two women and one man, recovered from their illnesses within two weeks of their mothers' deaths. The mothers had figured prominently in their children's delusions. Like many other surviving children, these patients failed to connect their improvement to their parents' deaths. Like Princess Maria, all three had previously "failed to emancipate themselves from [parental] domination." They all remained well at follow-up and lived normal lives. Perusal of hospital records revealed numerous similar cases, none of which was ever reported in the literature. The authors concluded, tartly and tellingly, that "maternal death apparently made adaptation to reality more inviting."

You don't have to be psychotic or even have a mother who drove you crazy only figuratively to respond to reality's invitation to live your own life after she dies.

Dialogue with the Dead

As the number of baby boomers losing their parents reaches critical mass, death is finally beginning to get its due. After decades of avoidance, a radically new approach that challenges the traditional understanding of mourning and its aftermath is good news; it makes death benefits easier to grasp and to achieve.

Leaving the deceased behind used to be considered the primary task of grieving. In his 1917 essay "Mourning and Melancholia," Freud wrote that the bereaved must sever their ties to the dead to be able to love again; he believed that emotional energy cannot be invested in a new relationship until it is first disconnected from an old one and that the ability to do so differentiates healthy mourning from neurotic "melancholia" (depression). Contemporary grief counselors have perpetuated the notion that survivors need to detach in order to restore emotional equilibrium, and mental health is still measured by the degree of separation they achieve.

But psychoanalysis has changed profoundly in the ninety years since Freud's essay; attention has now shifted from internal psychological processes to relationships. As a result, therapists increasingly focus on how to maintain meaningful connections with the dead (particularly with dead parents) rather than primarily on how to detach from them and return to the emotional status quo. Whatever the nature of the bond, parents never leave us; after death they simply move their residence from the outer world to the inner and accompany us for the rest of our lives. The relationship is just as real when it exists exclusively within our psyches—but then it belongs to us alone and is ours to alter. Therefore, we can do more than merely return to where and what we were before our loss; we can go forward.

The death of parents ushers in a second identity crisis. We revisit the same issues we struggled with the first time around—autonomy versus connection—with a more fully formed personality, more life experience, and a more solid place in the world.

Mourning looks very different from this perspective; it is not a time-limited, linear progression of universal stages but rather an idiosyncratic process that is ongoing, episodic, and fluid. Its function is to console and strengthen the self. Buried memories resurface when we least expect them; years do not loosen the links to the past. A recent study of 220 bereaved adults showed that the intensity of their feelings about their parents, rather than how long they had been dead—or even how much time they had spent with their parents when they were alive—determined the length and depth of their grief. Another researcher found only a "negligible" difference in the potency of the parent/child bond between adults whose parents were alive and those whose parents were long dead. Since parents are always psychically available, we have infinite opportunities to reinvent them, and ourselves.

Deceased mothers and fathers live on in their children's minds, but with a crucial, and helpful, difference: all further communication with them is unilateral, which makes it much easier to understand. You have far more control over relationships with dead parents than with live ones—especially when a parent is as compelling a presence as my own mother was. Finally, as I myself discovered, you can pick and choose among legacies of character as well as possessions.

Bereavement, we now know, is an active and creative state of mind, not simply a trauma to be passively endured. Working through the loss of any parent requires excruciatingly painful, but ultimately rewarding, mental effort—over decades, not months. As a result, there is far more room for exercising will in renegotiating posthumous relationships than anyone realized. And it is a process that can begin at any time.

Griefwork, the conscious and unconscious process of dealing with a death, actually keeps mourners healthy because it allows them to defy the helplessness of loss. This explains why the majority of adults who lose a parent do not become depressed or suffer other long-term emotional problems. The resulting feeling of mastery also breeds benefits.

The changes that death makes possible run the gamut from subtle shifts in feeling that nobody else notices to dramatic actions that no stranger could miss. Every change reflects modifications in the inner dialogue with a dead parent; identity, autonomy, and perspective are the topics we "discuss" with them for the rest of our lives.

Immediately after the funeral, many adults feel closer to the lost parent than they have in years, no matter how ambivalent their attachment; this was certainly true in my case. Even though the last few years of my mother's life had been anything but easy for me, I remember feeling strangely comforted by the memorial candle that burned for a week after she died, as though the flame were her spirit, and I dreaded the moment it would be extinguished and she would vanish from the world. Survivors often express their connection by "catching" the symptoms of a parent's final illness; immediately after my mother's fatal heart attack, I anxiously attended to the beating of my own heart as though her fate must be mine—a feeling both alien (I had no cardiac problem) and compelling. The primitive fusion that this physical empathy embodies is the precursor to sorting out what belongs to whom and eventually integrating selected traits of the parent's personality into an expanded identity, something that can and should be done consciously and systematically.

As we struggle to come to terms, dreams about parents, including scenes from years ago, suddenly reappear; they are a priceless tool for discovering death benefits. The unconscious doesn't make clear distinctions between past and present or living and dead;

people often receive phone calls from the dead in their dreams, and although I haven't lived with my parents since 1965, I still sometimes give their long-disconnected phone number instead of my own. While I was writing this book, I placed a catalog order by telephone from my home in New York City, and the operator asked me where I was calling from. "Cincinnati, Ohio," I instantly replied; of course, it was true. In mourning our parents we also mourn (and return to) our lost childhood.

Many surviving children not only hold onto a parental possession after its owner dies but also make it symbolically their own by transforming it. A woman I interviewed converted her mother's diamond ring into a necklace of her own design, and one of my patients reframed a painting of his father's. In addition to fitting my mother's highly charged red sunglasses with new lenses, I took an unusual carved picture frame of hers and replaced the print that had always been in it with one I preferred.

Losing your first parent makes you half an orphan; the painful recognition that hits you after burying your second is that you're nobody's child anymore. This automatic, unsolicited promotion to the older generation is also expressed somatically. I suddenly felt older and unwittingly began thinking of myself—and even referring to myself—as the age I would be on my next birthday rather than the age I was. The skin on my face, which could hardly have changed from the day before, seemed more wrinkled, my hair a little grayer. No one saw these signs but me.

As alive as it was for me, my childhood simultaneously seemed further away as soon as both my parents were gone. I found the extra distance enlightening as well as sobering, because, with no conscious effort on my part, there was suddenly a new depth to my thinking about the past. To my surprise, my father—who had been dead for twenty-five years—came into focus as well as my mother. Even though I had written three books in which they appeared, now I found I had gained new access into both my parents' interior lives. What, I wondered, must my mother and father have gone through when they were my age? It struck me how sad and frightened my father must have been, how desperate my mother must have felt, how neither of them had any idea what to do. I understood that what at the time seemed like callous unconcern for me was unbearable, blinding, and uncontrollable preoccupation with themselves. As a middle-aged woman familiar with limitations and remorse, theirs no longer shocked or outraged me. Sympathy and empathy for their failings—failings that had caused me anguish that had never fully healed—came naturally. I was without them, I had become them, and I could finally see them.

I also found myself thinking about how each of them dealt with illness and faced death, seeking something to console or assist or inspire me when my own time came. This was harder to do with my father, who died when I was much younger and less aware. I was estranged from him then, to my eternal regret, and therefore unable either to help him or communicate with him, but I know that he loved me to the end despite his terror, pain, and despair. I was able to recover and incorporate the professional calm and expertise he displayed in emergencies, the legacy of his medical training. Released from the burden of managing my mother's last years, I was flooded with admiration for her gallantry, how she maintained not only her dignity but her vitality until the last moment of consciousness. I hope I inherited some of her gumption and that I can draw on it when I need it. I expect to do more thinking about them as I age, finding aspects of each one to emulate and to avoid.

We need to take yet another step in reconsidering mourning: resurrecting and redefining, rather than discarding, the significance of detaching from the dead. Paradoxically, detachment is an integral part of the mature posthumous bond an adult maintains with a parent. It helps us uncover the essence of the relationship beyond the noise of interaction. I believe that what we disconnect from, if we are lucky and effective mourners, is not the relationship with deceased parents per se but rather the way we were embedded in that relationship when they were alive. This new stance permits us to reinterpret the past, and expands our understanding of who our parents were and who we were in relation to them, enhancing recognition, compassion, and sympathy for all concerned. This type of detachment radically changed my life, and the lives of the people I interviewed, for the better. When we finally see with adult eyes, we can recover as well as discover our parents' hidden strengths and discard their newly obvious weaknesses. Detachment, the perspective it affords, and the growth it makes possible, is the greatest death benefit of all, and the prerequisite for all the rest.

CHAPTER 3

GOING THROUGH THE STUFF

Choosing a Legacy

❧

I've gone through my family's "stuff" five times so far—twice in dwellings in the last seven years (first I dismantled the contents of my parents' house when my mother moved out, then I took a few last things from her assisted-living apartment when she died), and twice in dreams two or more years later. Taking a psychological inventory of my mother's character when I wrote this book was my most recent attempt. I'm not done yet; I intend to keep doing it for the rest of my life.

Although we cannot pick our parents, we can have considerable say in which of their attributes get the most weight after they die. Mindfully deciding among their belongings is the first opportunity to make that choice. Happily, the process can be revisited internally long after the house is sold, the memorabilia reviewed, the valuables procured, and the unwanted contents given away.

Sorting through parents' possessions and deciding what to keep and what to discard is one of the first duties after they die and a potent metaphor for the psychological work ahead. Everybody dreads the onerous task and the host of anxieties—childhood memories, intimations of mortality, sibling rivalry, unfinished business—it inevitably generates. As a patient of mine put it,

> What of my mother do I want to take with me? Her possessions are all that's left of her life, and I hate to give anything away, because she treasured it. Certain core things are so much a part of her that I can't imagine actually owning them; it moves me up a generation. Doing this puts her in a different context—in my past, and less in my present. Now she's somebody who had an influence, not somebody I'm working around.

How a person goes about the selection process is revealing. Some pick and choose over a few days, trying to make a rational, or at least equitable, distribution among siblings. Some spend months carefully sifting through every item in the household inventory, unable to throw anything away—incorporating, rather than integrating, a parent's life.

Too many people simply relegate objects to permanent psychic as well as physical storage, never engaging with their parents' possessions or consciously addressing what they want or how they feel. One man I know crammed everything within arm's reach into a suitcase and left town in four hours, effectively (he thought) slamming the door on his parents and his past. Another acquaintance of mine left his mother's estate in suspended animation, refusing even to enter his childhood home—let alone decide what he wanted—for two years. He was waiting, he explained, until he had "absorbed" her death; in actuality, he was denying its impact, as well as avoiding any conflict with his rapacious relatives. A pair of sisters let their father's weekend house lay fallow for seven years, occasionally removing a few artifacts, until they could bring themselves to empty the place. This was the only way they could process his slow, painful demise.

Many adults begin sorting scrupulously, hoping to create order or find meaning, but quickly become inundated and end up dumping the undigestible detritus. A fastidious son (a historian, not surprisingly) recalled his experience in a letter he wrote to me:

> The Smith family are keepers (I came upon a stack of receipts neatly tied in twine labeled "Oats For Penelope." Penelope was the chestnut mare that pulled my grandfather's buggy when he was starting out as a doctor in Sacramento), and at first I examined every scrap of paper as though it were the Rosetta Stone. Soon enough, though, the exercise felt like one of desperation, as if I were jettisoning broken lamps and Salton hot trays into black waters that were rising about a foundering ship.

Irony masked the anxiety and rage he felt at being saddled with a responsibility he could never adequately discharge—a position his father (and his father before him) had put him in all his life. He himself was the ship foundering under the weight of unacknowledged resentment and obligation.

The wisest and most productive way to go through stuff—your parents' physical possessions initially and their psychological legacy later on—is to take your time but not too much time. Be serious, systematic, and aware of the import of the task while recognizing that it cannot, and need not, be done perfectly.

What an heir does with the chosen possessions is telling. Two women, both high school teachers, had dramatically different ways of dealing with the furniture and jewelry they inherited from mothers who had loomed too large. Cindy Atkins plunked the unedited belongings in her living room like august alien presences, preserving her mother's emotional legacy as imperviously as her antimacassars:

> I love Victoriana, and that's what she had, so I took more of the family furniture than anybody else. My house is like a museum. I never touch the stuff—it's just there.

Beth Grant used another strategy, making it her business to "touch the stuff," and working hard to find the right place for her mother's lamps, rugs, and paintings. She felt triumphant at the result of her mental and physical labor:

> I'm really enjoying my apartment because I integrated her things so seamlessly. It looks more complete and changed now—I'm thrilled to see my new living room. A lot of it's hers, but it's very much me.

For two years both of them kept their mothers' lavish diamonds in safety deposit boxes—perhaps unconsciously to reassure themselves that the original owners really were dead and the treasures legitimately theirs. Even then Cindy could not lay direct claim to her inheritance, but she came up with a novel compromise solution:

I could never wear her ring because if I lost it she'd have been right when she said, "You're always careless; I can't give you anything, you'll just destroy it." Then I bought an imitation diamond ring that looked just like hers for $100. I don't wear it on my ring finger. It's a good-luck token for me because I know I can always buy another one. This jewelry is the only way my mother is present in my life.

Cindy's mother is actually present in her life in a far more central and destructive way than the accusatory ring her daughter dares not wear; her critical attitude continues to define Cindy's self-image as untrustworthy and undeserving. "I hoped my mother's death would make a difference," she observed, "and in some ways it didn't." By addressing the power she attributes to the ring, Cindy could begin to create even better luck for herself: the positive difference a mother's death can make. Any son or daughter who seeks but does not receive death benefits should ask why not. Unfinished business with the parent is often the obstacle.

After a decent interval had elapsed, Beth was ready to revisit her mother's legacy and treat the ring as she had the furniture, integrating it into her own world and altering it to her own taste. She, too, could not wear the stone that once adorned her mother's finger—but it was a wish for self-expression rather than fear of the consequences that prevented her:

I decided to take my mother's two-carat diamond ring out of the vault; it finally felt right to make it mine and not feel guilty. But I couldn't just wear her ring—it wouldn't be me—so I had a jeweler redesign it as a necklace. The easiest thing would have been to hang it off a chain as is, but I

didn't want to do that either. I needed to make something
different out of it.

Beth's mother's ring is not the only thing she is redesigning to
her own specifications; she is making something different of and
for herself.

The relationship each of these women is negotiating with her
dead mother is reflected in the role she assigns to possessions.
One maintains her mother as an internal critic and inhibiting
presence; the other is breaking free.

Active self-reflection plays a far greater role than we realize in
shaping an emotional inheritance. Inordinate guilt, greed, reflex-
ive repudiation, or being in too much of a hurry for "closure"—as
though we can ever be done with our own history—when selecting heirlooms can limit success the first time around, but there are
plenty of other chances. There's always more stuff to go through
and more life experience to bring to the process.

Based on my own experience, I offer the following guidelines
for conducting the most fruitful emotional inventory:

Going Through the (Psychological) Stuff

- Use the physical inventory you took as a reference point
  for the psychological one to follow; the experiences and
  memories a parent's possessions and the artifacts of
  childhood evoked can lead you to understand your
  parent's character and its impact on your own. Expect
  emotions even more intense and contradictory when
  conducting the psychological inventory than when
  conducting the physical one.

Four Questions for Conducting Your Psychological Inventory

1. What did you get from your parent that you want to keep?
2. What did your parent have that you didn't get and that you regret missing?
3. What did you get from your parent that you want to discard?
4. What did you need that your parent couldn't provide?

- Take the stance of a historian or researcher when documenting the story of your parent's life and reconsidering your own past in the process. Your goal is to broaden your appreciation and understanding of your parent and yourself. A deeply considered, healthily detached history is the best foundation for the next step—a detailed emotional survey.

- Consider other points of view than your own; what you hear from people in your parents' lives may be a revelation.

- Psychological inventories take time. Go through a conscious selection process; don't simply keep everything or throw everything away. Neither wholesale repudiation nor wholesale incorporation of a parent's emotional legacy promotes integration and change. What you choose to leave behind can be as important as what you take.

- Expect to have regrets about what you failed to receive and what you got that you didn't want. There is no perfect closure, or perfect continuity, in relationships with parents; they are always works in progress.

※

Constructing a positive legacy from a problematic parent is a special skill. Some people seem to have a knack for going through their parents' characters the same way they go through their closets—keeping what they want and leaving the rest behind. It is striking how often they use the word "choice" in describing their efforts to discover and hold onto the best (and sometimes the only good thing) their parents had to offer.

Aaron Goodman's father was a psychiatrist with an international reputation for wisdom as well as brilliance, but the private man his son knew was an irresponsible, intimidating misogynist. Still, strangers lowered their voices when they sang his praises. "I was his goodwill ambassador to the world," said Aaron bitterly of the monumental figure whose attention he could never hold and who cast an impossibly long shadow. Aaron considered his father's death a year earlier, at age eighty-nine, an opportunity to assess his intellectual and emotional heritage. "For the first time I can decide not only how I want to live but who I am," he said. "My purpose is to give myself the power to choose which parts of him I want to keep and which to jettison." So far, he has decided to "keep his profession, and jettison his attitude toward women."

Diane Gordon thought of her imposing mother "as a Sherman tank or a mother tigress, depending on whether she was coming at you or defending you." She felt so scrutinized that, although a professional chef herself, she never dared cook in her mother's kitchen; "one of her was quite enough," she said, with mingled admiration and relief. But Diane has managed to deemphasize the tank and concentrate on the tigress. She picks the memories to focus on and identify with:

> In high school I wanted to take a schedule of advanced courses that wouldn't allow me to have lunch, and the counselor wouldn't approve it. My mother was home making garlic pickles. Without washing her hands, she drove off with me. She swept into the counselor's office—she was an English professor with a phenomenal vocabulary and she was waving her hands around a lot. Between the garlic and the force of my mother's personality, the counselor was backed against the wall, and I got the schedule changed that day. I too am a fighter; I discovered that I can channel my inner tiger. What I choose to have her leave me is her protection and love.

Even when the emotional "estate" a parent bequeaths is mixed or the material one meager, a child can still seek what was best and cling to it. Diane selected the "fierceness of her [mother's] devotion," not her "cutting remarks," to "think of as being core." Similarly, playwright David Schwartz decided to be inspired by his mother's musical talent rather than repelled by her miserliness; piano scores were the only possessions of hers he deemed worth keeping.

Psychological housecleaning does not come easily for most people. It takes determination and a lot of practice to develop the requisite nonpunitive self-awareness as well as the ability to take stock periodically and edit the way our parents live on in us. This process, of course, is not entirely conscious—or else we would not so often notice with dismay (or have it pointed out to us by spouses) that we are "just like" the worst aspects of our forebears. So many of our parents' attributes are absorbed unawares that we often feel more chosen than choosing. But thinking about what we retain makes a difference; it gives us some say. The son of an alcoholic, for example, need not become one himself if he unflinchingly identifies the trait, considers its impact on him as a child, and manages it as an adult, any more than a daughter has to express anger by flying into the same destructive rages her mother did and blaming her own children as she herself was blamed. Recognition is the key. It creates receptivity and offers ourselves material to ponder subliminally, where the deepest changes originate. Like objects in the household inventory, character traits must be scrutinized to determine which to emulate, which to extirpate, and which to renovate.

Going through the stuff can change your life. Seemingly insignificant artifacts found by chance among a parent's belongings often provide unimagined benefits to a grieving child—or to an aggrieved one. Strands of hair and tattered sheets of paper with fading ink offer consolation and longed-for explanations for hurts that seemed impossible to heal. When a photographer who had been estranged from her mother for years found a locket on the table beside the deathbed containing her own hair, she realized that, despite the enmity between them, she had never totally lost her mother's love. An accompanist rummaging through her mother's papers discovered a diary entry her mother had made as a young girl, before life had hardened her into the cold, violent woman who haunted her daughter's nightmares:

> She'd written, "Oh Life, please bring me happiness." I never knew her as happy, only angry. I welcome seeing a totally different side. I always felt bad because I thought I was responsible for her happiness. In death I'm sorry; now I wish I could have.

Becoming acquainted with the hopeful, spirited adolescent who had written those words permitted her to grieve for her mother's sorrow and to appreciate her. Consoled herself, she wished she could have consoled. Eventually her nightmares were transformed into dreams of mutual goodwill.

Jan Kahn's mother stopped speaking to her twenty-six-year-old daughter when Jan told her she was gay; only a diagnosis of terminal cancer two years later made her relent. "She wanted me back in her life on a 'Don't Ask/Don't Tell' basis," Jan recalled, and they reconciled on her mother's terms because "her suffering was so horrific that the issue faded to the sidelines." Though Jan never stopped longing for her mother's blessing, it was never forthcoming. "At the very end when we started to get close I broached the subject and she froze up—it was clear that those were the boundaries." The pain of her mother's rejection coupled with the agony of her death left her daughter doubly bereft and drove anger as well as grief underground.

Only after her father died five years later could she bring herself to open her mother's jewelry box. "A friend who loved costume jewelry was coming to town, and I thought there might be something she'd like," she explained. Among the baubles lay something priceless and utterly unexpected:

> As I'm going through it I find a note. Her penmanship showed she must have written it at the very end of her life—the writing was very shaky and up and down and it used to be perfect. It said, "Dear Jan, I'm sorry for any hurt and pain I have ever caused you." I was devastated: I felt heard.

❧

Recently, Beth Grant found some more of her parents' stuff to go through. Perhaps because she'd been so successful at integrating the furniture and the jewelry, her psyche presented another, even more basic, batch of it for her consideration in a dream:

> I was looking for closet space and found an extra room in my house that I didn't realize was there. Then I saw that I had suitcases full of my father's and mother's clothes. I had to clean it up before I could use the room—it hadn't been done when they died. It was going to be a big job, but then I'd have room for all my own stuff.

Until she gets rid of her parents' "baggage," there will not be enough room for the newly expansive self that Beth is creating; she is studying acting in middle age and hopes to pursue a second career on the stage. Now is the time to discard her parents' confining and outmoded clothes—the roles they ordained for her—and play the roles she chooses for herself. The dream says her work is cut out for her and that she will have a room of her own as her reward.

Like Beth, I, too, was confronted with more stuff to sort through on the second anniversary of my mother's death, a typical time for reassessing one's inheritance. I, too, had done a thorough job initially; I'd made my selection attentively, given friends the things I wouldn't use, fitted her Navajo rugs around my own kilims—even reacquisitioned gifts I'd given her—with gratitude and without guilt. Then a dream told me that I wasn't finished, either, and showed me what I had to confront.

I dreamed I was back in my mother's house. Most of the contents were gone, but several strange new things had taken their place. On a (nonexistent) patio I found two neglected potted plants, a fern with frozen fronds that had been left out in the cold and a tree that had lost most of its leaves because it hadn't been watered. Both would be inconvenient to take with me. I could defrost the fern and water the tree and hope new leaves would sprout; was trying to revive them worth the effort? There was no clear resolution in the dream.

Then I went inside where a gigantic, tacky print of a Frida Kahlo painting now took up an entire wall; this I definitely didn't want. On the way out I noticed a garish old plastic wall clock, its hands stuck at 11:30. Should I take it anyway? I knew it couldn't be fixed, and after a short debate with myself, I left it on the wall.

As I was leaving, I saw that the people next door were moving out, and strangers were moving in. Nothing was still the same. Closing the door on everything I found there felt irrevocable and necessary, as if I were closing a chapter of my life.

The three objects in the dream—the plants, the painting, and the clock—represent my mother's most problematic qualities. Dreaming about them was the beginning of my taking inventory of her character and understanding her impact on me, which took me the next year to accomplish, and which became the basis of my death benefit.

I shunned the cheap Frida Kahlo reproduction, discarding for good my identification with the side of my mother who, like the Mexican artist, often acted like an exhibitionistic masochist and who never left her unfaithful husband. Her pessimism is represented by the old clock that only shows the eleventh hour, an attitude that still beckons even though I fight it. When I accept that time isn't always running out and catastrophe isn't always just around the corner, I can get myself a new clock—one that shows me that I have more time and more possibilities than she did.

What about the frozen and desiccated plants? These represent my mother's coldness and periodic inability to take care of me emotionally, as well as my own response to her. When I had this dream, I was struggling to determine whether my love and sense of her as my inconsistent but mostly well-meaning nurturer could be revived, a question I was able to answer in a way that changed my life; the issue was unresolved in the dream because I hadn't tackled it yet. This was a preview of coming attractions.

When I awoke, I discovered that my living potted fig tree, which I had in fact taken in from the cold months earlier, had put forth a tiny leaf in the dead of winter. I took it as a good omen, and it was.

Leaving my mother's world, even the parts that drove me crazy, unsettles me and makes me feel adrift. Maybe one reason we hold onto and embody so much of our parents' characters, including traits we despise, is that it's the only way we know to maintain a tie to them. You can't let the bad parts go until you understand why they had those qualities and that you don't have to keep them.

Parents' material legacies are resonant and numinous, alive with their presence and our memories. These objects evoke not only the personalities and tastes of their original owners but also the first world we knew. New facets emerge as our relationship with them evolves, some of which take considerable time and distance to appear. New "stuff" always presents itself, along with new ways to "go through" it.

The ritual of picking and pitching the family tchotchkes is not a onetime event that ends when the Salvation Army truck arrives. It is the first installment of an enterprise that lasts a lifetime: posthumously assimilating and re-creating parents. Going through the stuff is where death benefits begin.

PART II

LIFE BENEFITS

Body, Mind, and Spirit

CHAPTER 4

USING THE GOOD CHINA

Deserving a Life at Last

჻

The pursuit of happiness may be an inalienable right, but many people cannot claim it until their parents are gone. Only then do they feel that life's joys—freedom, children, sexual pleasure, cherished possessions, a home of one's own—are legitimately theirs. Guilt gets in the way, or growing up in a culture of deprivation. For some, simply surviving takes all their energy, leaving none for expansiveness. Very often, in ways that astonish the celebrant, death brings a license to live.

Jane Greenberg's fairy tale world—she was the daughter of a Hollywood mogul—disintegrated when she was fifteen years old. In rapid succession, her mother died of cancer, her father went AWOL, and in a fit of jealous rage her mentally ill older brother destroyed everything her mother had left her. There was no stuff for her to go through—no photographs, no jewelry, no mementos of any kind—and no way to process her losses. As a consequence Jane spent her early adulthood maintaining the protective conviction that she had no right to anything precious; if she deserved nothing, it didn't matter that she had nothing. She eventually moved from the now-desolate Brentwood mansion to a small, bare-bones apartment in Chicago; never married; and devoted herself to her career as a reporter. Only when her father died thirty years later was she able to recover sustaining memories and the right to the good things in life.

"My orientation was always 'the sky's gonna fall,'" Jane recalled, "but now I feel more optimistic; I've become an optimistic pessimist." She attributes this subtle but radical change in attitude to insights into her father's character made possible by his death: "Now I have back all the great stuff about him. A flood of memories—how funny and creative he was—came rushing back; all the rage has melted away."

Even before tragedy struck their family, Mr. Greenberg's larger-than-life presence dominated everything and everybody around him; "I didn't have to see *The Producers*," his daughter observed, "I lived it." Insecurity masked by grandiosity compelled him to grab the spotlight and left his daughter nothing but a supporting role; he destroyed his son, whom he perceived as a rival, by denying him any role at all. He swept Jane off to Paris for a weekend when she was thirty-eight, but he could never acknowledge her accomplishments, nor appreciate her quirky looks or her dark humor. "He had such a profound need to be the center of the world that he couldn't let anybody in, so I always came up short," she said. "While he was alive I never felt pretty, never knew that he was proud of me, but now I do; this transition has allowed me to know." As her rage melted, her sense of doom and disenfranchisement dissipated as well.

When death forced her father offstage, Jane became the star of her own life. She and the (quiet, retiring) man she'd met at age forty moved in together. Two years later, she adopted a baby girl—something precious that was truly hers. Miraculously, she retrieved what she thought she had lost forever. "Having Susie brings my father back in a weird way. When I look at her, I see him looking at her, making a silly face. He's a flirt—I hear his voice. He's right here looking at her; all this I see." Now a loving mother herself, the tender scene she conjures allows her to recover her parents and the best of her own childhood.

Love and pride revived Jane's long-buried taste for beautiful things. "I always had a sense of rehearsal, that you're saving your good stuff for later. Now I realize I should use the good china—I should go for it." The metaphorical china wasn't all she deserved to enjoy; she wanted real napkins and tablecloths, too: "I love vintage linen. I used to keep it all in tissue paper, but I'm starting to use it, trying to live a little bit more in the moment."

Jane weathered a recent loss without forfeiting her ability to treat herself well; even getting laid off was more manageable in her father's absence. "If this had happened when he was alive it would have been much more traumatic; if I lost a job he lost a job. I would have taken his disappointment and anger on myself to protect him from a sense of personal injury. With him gone it ended up not being so bad. I don't know if it's possible to be completely resolved about a parent's death, but I've come close. I feel pretty good where I am." At last, the banquet of life is hers to savor.

⁓

Depressed mothers may be less obviously overwhelming than grandiose fathers, but they take up as much psychic room. Most children secretly feel liberated when death lifts their oppression, although few can cheerfully admit it. Only a handful believe their parents would actually approve.

Iris Connor is overjoyed that her own depression dissipated after her mother died, but people are scandalized when she says so—even though she knows her mother would be delighted. "Soon after her funeral, I was sitting on a couch with a friend who offered condolences, and I said, 'Thank you, but you know, I'm free to be happy now.' He was shocked because he was close to his mother." Iris had felt closed in by hers. "Her view of the world affected my view," she said. She'd always felt guilty, responsible for her mother's happiness but unable to bring it about. "Nothing was ever enough for her. If I came for a weekend she asked why it wasn't three days. I grew up afraid. She's like a virus—she walks into the room and you catch it." A depressive parent breeds pessimism in a child just like a narcissistic one does, because you can't fill the void for either one. Jane, the mogul's daughter, expected the sky to fall any minute; Iris remembers "always waiting for the other shoe to drop; it's the biggest thing I've had to overcome."

Since her mother's death, Iris's self-blame has vanished. "This is my epiphany," she says, with unconcealed joy. "She really did drain me of energy—now I've got more of it for myself and for the world. I don't worry about being depressed anymore. I don't think that will ever happen again. I've got no guilt, not a shred. I'm an orphan but I'm stronger than ever being alone, stronger and less afraid."

What enables Iris to escape feeling wretched for the rest of her life, unable to forgive herself for not healing her mother—or her mother for demanding that she do so? Why isn't she compelled to punish herself by remaining her mother's companion in misery? Her conviction that her mother wished her well even though she could never say so directly. Like the gleam that Jane imagines in her father's eye as he looks at his granddaughter, Iris feels her mother's joy that her daughter is happier than she was herself—an indication of real devotion. Both women absolve their parents of blame because death makes it possible for them to know that they were loved. "She'd be the first to say she's glad—she'd be so pleased that I'm not plagued the way she was; she didn't mean to hold me down." Iris's mother gives her more now than she could when she was alive. Whenever there is love to recover from the dead, the living should seek to retrieve it; the good memories can sustain you and drive out the bad ones. "I know she loved me but it was imperfect, as those things are," Iris declares. "She did want the best. I've got a clear-eyed view of who she was, and I appreciate what she gave me, how free she was with hugs and compliments. She never said an unkind thing to me and was generous with support—I have to give her credit, even though it was not helpful that she worried and passed that on." Death cleared Iris's vision, cured her "virus," and revealed that she deserved the best of everything. With her mother's blessing, she declares, "I'm unstoppable."

Sometimes what a child really needs is skin deep—as Molly Talbot found when she was "seized" with the impulse to buy a sexy wig after her father died, laying claim to her femininity and her right to be noticed. "It was almost like possession," she said. "I wanted suddenly to have long hair, so I took the money my aunt gave me the week after he died and went to Macy's and bought it." Voluptuous tresses were a very charged commodity in Molly's family; her "autocratic, obnoxious" father forbade it, and Molly's mother considered her daughter's coiffure inferior because it did not resemble her own. ("She'd had golden curls as a child. She used to tell me, 'Your brothers got the good hair.'")

Going out and getting good hair of her own choosing was the first time she dared to draw attention to herself. "I didn't come into my sexual own until my father died," she said. "I'd been very repressed, and wore only black." When he was no longer around to disapprove, life got more colorful. Her mother died years later, and Molly was "seized" all over again; this time, she had to pierce her ears. "It was my way of decorating myself, making myself more alluring— with her gone I could enjoy myself. That put the dot on the 'i' of my emancipation." Molly's mother had been fond of quoting Thoreau's maxim, "Most men live lives of quiet desperation"; "What a goal for your daughter!" Molly exclaimed, when she realized she had been given a prescription rather than a warning. Her new hair and earrings were her weapons of hope and desire as she went out into the world, defying resignation, depression, and defeat.

❧

Houses are powerful symbols; in dreams they stand for our bodies, our psyches, and our selves. Havens or prisons, they can be venues for building a foundation and living to the hilt, or receptacles for childhood experiences best left behind.

"I want to own some ground before I'm in it," announced David Schwartz. His mother's unnecessary self-deprivations in the last years of her life, and her desolate death, galvanized him to look for property in the country and to purchase a cabin on twenty-two acres the day he saw it. Witnessing the deadening effects of his parents' miserliness made him a passionate advocate of living to the fullest.

Although comfortably middle class, the Schwartzes never allowed themselves good china, or nice clothes, or even proper medical care when it became necessary; limiting expenditures and prematurely divesting themselves of possessions were ways to maintain control when they felt it slipping away. "I'd been very distressed by things my mother gave away, like the pinball machine they had in the basement," her son said. "My father got this crazy notion that they had to get rid of it because they might move, and she went along although she liked playing it. This was folly in the guise of planning, dying in the guise of planning. I thought it was a terrible idea—how much would it have cost to remove the thing when the time came?" He saw that his parents were protecting themselves preemptively against loss ("If you destroy it you can't lose it"), but he also saw the cost. "They gave up. What good does the giving up do you? I didn't want to be ruled by fears pretending to be prudence. Fears prevent you from living." David's decision to buy a place of his own signaled his disentanglement from his mother's view of the world and asserted his identity as a competent adult who could take healthy risks.

David and his wife had considered buying a retreat years earlier, but the prospect of renovating and maintaining it had seemed beyond him. "We'd had all these worries about a house we looked at that had a bathroom I couldn't stand up in. Then it felt like such a daunting thing to do—so many unknowns, so many responsibilities—but this time I decided to screw it; we actually ended up ripping out the bathroom of this house and starting from scratch. You take on a bunch of problems, but so what? You get the satisfaction of solving them. You might as well say if you have a hand you'll have to keep washing it, you'll have to cut the nails, you could hit it—all true, but should you not have a hand because of that? I became a property owner like my parents, but in a joyous way. My mother's death broke a spell, broke my malignant identification with stasis."

To buy a home of one's own is to have a place in the world, to find stability comforting rather than claustrophobic, and to believe in the future. Sandy Johnson couldn't imagine feeling any of those things until she saw her father on his deathbed.

This fifty-one-year-old executive quaked as she approached his hospital room; a quarter century had passed since she'd had contact with the alcoholic brute who had abandoned his family. "When my aunt called and told me that he was dying, I was terrified," she said. "I knew I had to see him, but I didn't know what he would do to me—and then I saw that he was just a weak, frail old man."

As scared as she was of him, Sandy never ceased longing for her father. His presence was a constant menace, but she was his favorite, the only one in the family whom he neither beat nor molested. "I loved my dad—he was my dad; we used to go sailing together. He had terrible parts but he was extremely intelligent. Of all the siblings, I was the one who held off hating him the most. I identified with him, and even called the angry part of myself 'George'—my father's name." Although Sandy got the best he had to offer, she paid a price for her loyalty ("I've never been successful in an intimate relationship") and blamed herself that he abandoned her.

Sandy's reaction to her father's death (he was already unconscious when she arrived) amazed her. "It was the funniest thing—he passed away and all of a sudden I felt lighthearted. I realized that my entire life I'd been looking around every corner for a monster to snatch me—and then my fear was gone. I hadn't known how on guard I was or how much I loved him. His death was a turning point." She and her younger sister, whom she had taken along for this final encounter, also had the remarkable luck of speaking to a priest who had spent time with their father in the hospital. They learned that he died grief-stricken and remorseful.

"He was a destroyed man. I see that he wasn't capable and it isn't my fault," Sandy said, her relief palpable.

The experience transformed her from a nomad into a homeowner. "I had never bought a house; the longest I'd lived in a rented apartment was three years. I had no roots anywhere because I had to keep moving. I think I was running from him; finally I can stop." She can stay put because she also stopped running from her inner "George." "I never thought I deserved anything in life—I thought I must have been a rotten person or he wouldn't have left," she said. Sandy's newborn sense of entitlement permitted her to create a real home for herself, the first she ever had, and to flourish there. "I'm no longer on hold—I'm free to go on with my life. I was stuck before, always on the edge; now I let my emotions flow. If I'm sad, I cry." Now that she is rooted, she can grow.

A parent's death earns many adults the right to have a home and the possessions to fill it. But for some people, deserving life means mobility rather than stability—the freedom to go wherever they please. Marsha Montgomery's act of liberation after both her parents died was buying a one-way ticket to Rome. For the first time in her life, there was nobody she had to take care of, so when her husband got an offer to relocate for three years, she told him to grab it. "At last nothing was tying me down," she said. "I'd had a diabetic mother since age twenty, and when she died five years ago my debilitated father moved in with us, so I've always felt I needed to stay around. I was so tied up in their health and well-being that my own slipped, mentally and physically." Marsha spent her young adulthood enslaved by their demands. "My relationship with my mother was always parent and child reversed, even before she became ill," she said. "She'd call in a panic in the middle of the night and say, 'You've got to come over. I can't breathe.' It would be horrible not to go. I'd be on my way, and she'd ask, 'Why aren't you here yet?' It didn't matter how much I did. Her death brought me relief and guilt that I felt relief."

Taking care of her father when he moved in was just as all-consuming. She remembers sitting in her driveway after work and dreading going inside because she couldn't bear to assume the roles of cook, nurse, and cheerleader. She had internalized these expectations to such an extent that she never considered the noxious impact of his presence on her marriage or her life; the only indication of her true feelings was a vivid dream that he was a misshapen creature screaming at her for ignoring his "little monster needs." Houses and their desperate, selfish inhabitants bred claustrophobia, never comfort.

Therapists (myself included) frequently warn patients against the "geographic solution," arguing that moving to another place never solves anything because you can't help taking yourself along to the new location. But Marsha's situation is an exception; for her, moving was an act of assertion, not avoidance. It gave her room to think, to breathe, and to break away. "I was picking up and leaving a whole part of life that wasn't good and that had taken over my will," Marsha explained. "I felt absolutely free to do whatever I wanted, free of obligation and judgment. I could have adventures—I could get my whole body tattooed, or decide I want to smoke five packs a day, leave my husband tomorrow, join a rock band! I am now the keeper of my destiny, of how extraordinary or how pedestrian my life becomes."

When death breaks the spell of being imprisoned in a parent's world, it is cause for rejoicing.

CHAPTER 5

MY BODY, MYSELF

Health and Beauty Benefits

❧

To declare that a parent's death is good for your health sounds counterintuitive as well as outrageous. Mourners suffer by definition; distracted by grief, they forget to eat or care for themselves. Not only do they lose interest in the outside world, but everyone assumes they will forego attending to their own needs for a significant period of time—some religions actually require them to give up pleasures like buying clothes or attending parties for a year. So why do so many survivors, most of whom genuinely grieved when their parents died, look and feel better than they ever have before—and betray no guilt about saying so?

When asked about death benefits, taking better physical care of themselves was the one people mentioned most often. They volunteered statements like, "I lost weight," "I stopped smoking," "I joined a gym," and "I went to the dentist." They also claimed that they felt more attractive—prettier, more graceful, or more masculine. They showed it, too; I was struck by how chic a colleague of mine looked six months after she lost her severe and self-depriving mother, how svelte a friend became soon after the death of his disapproving father. Even those who highly esteemed their parents discarded bad habits or acquired new, good ones. I noticed that several acquaintances took up challenging physical activities (tango dancing, weight lifting, yoga) with seriousness and zest— as I did myself—without realizing what prompted their enthusiasm; I only recognized that my renewed involvement with swimming was an identification with my mother when she had been dead for a year. When a parent's death grants permission to prosper—or serves as a warning to avoid a premature demise—a child feels both justified and proud of making the effort.

Such changes are never merely cosmetic; they reflect profound emotional alterations in the sense of self and in the relationship to the deceased. Looking and feeling better means taking charge, growing up, standing up, and living it up.

Perhaps paying more attention to health is the easiest death benefit to admit because it seems both more superficial and more morally acceptable than feeling freer or happier, but it's actually no different. In both cases the survivor is implicitly saying, "You are dead, but I'm still alive—let me make the most of it."

~~~

Barbara Goldstein has struggled with weight all her life. "I was always labeled a klutz," she confessed. "Even after a successful marriage and years of therapy, I could never let myself feel really good and comfortable in my body; being fat was how I presented myself to the world." Part of Barbara's battle with her waistline was genetic, but another part was parental; both her father and her mother were uncomfortable when she slimmed down in her twenties. "I was my most glamorous then," she recalled at age fifty-six. "My father and I used to go shopping to buy presents for my mother. One time we met a client of his who thought I was his girlfriend, and he never took me again. It was always a complicated dance—not letting myself be too close to him, too pleasing to him, because it would provoke my mother's ire." Her need not to upset either parent was a more powerful motivation to put the weight back on than her longing to look good was to keep it off.

Barbara couldn't stay on a diet until her father died when she was fifty-four; his absence made it possible. Her attitude is different, too; now her effort is for herself alone. "I don't have to deal with the triangle anymore," she said. "This time I've kept at it. I exercise three times a week. I have a better sense about my body than I've ever had—that it's really strong and capable. I don't feel like a schlump anymore; I'm physically competent, perfect, and complete." Her pleasure in her body lets her show herself off and to enjoy the attention that she used to flee. "The exterior is extremely important in my family, and now I like mine. I've let my inner Jewish princess out."

Weight loss is a typical way for women to express their self-possession after demanding parents die. As a patient of mine said, with not-quite-believing delight, "Something very basic in how I interact with the world has changed; I've lost weight for the first time in my life, without really trying. I always thought of myself as fat when my parents were alive—it was incredible when I went to the normal-size department instead of the plus-size one for the first time and nobody said, 'What the hell are you doing here?'"

Barbara could not let herself lose weight until her father died; Ellen Wagner's father had to die before she could realize she didn't need to diet. Their fathers defined body image for both of them, and only as orphans could they define it for themselves.

Ellen, a painter and graphic designer, was never slim enough for her perfectionistic parent. Mr. Wagner, a high-school gym teacher and coach who was athletic all his life, criticized everything about his daughter, especially appearance. "He had a stern look—he'd give it and my blood turned to ice," Ellen said. She was so desperate for a positive response that she "was always hugging him and sitting on his lap," even until she was twenty years old. "I realized it kind of late," she noted. Ellen's supposed girth was a major source of—or excuse for—her father's negativity. He "had a thing about weight," and his cold silence when he scrutinized her made her feel so terrible that she ate nothing but toast for several months in order to attain a level of litheness that she hoped would please him—only to discover that he didn't notice; "I even failed at being anorectic," she said. That her mother never came to her aid reinforced her misery.

Only after her father died did Ellen, then forty-eight, figure out that his obsession with her physique when she was a young woman had an entirely different cause: "I think I was growing into a sensuality that disturbed him." Like Barbara's father, he blamed his daughter for his own discomfort, and like Barbara, Ellen blamed herself. It never occurred to her that she looked perfectly normal, and always had. Once she understood that her need to please him distorted her perception, weight never worried her again.

Body image problems related to parental attitudes are most common in women, but men are not exempt. A man's sense of masculinity can be just as undermined by his father's criticism, and he can feel just as liberated when the disapproving glances and caustic remarks cease.

Peter Sawyer always felt like a changeling in his family, and his father treated him like one. Son of a mechanically minded alcoholic factory worker, the aesthetic, intellectual boy felt "totally inept and humiliated. We spoke different languages. He talked about 'ohms and amps' and I didn't care about that. I was an anomaly to him, a strange kid he never imagined having." The only kind of "oms" that ever interested Peter were in the yoga chants he learned when he spent a year in India while he was in college.

Just as Ellen starved herself to make her body conform to her father's standards, Peter polished his shoes and pressed and laid out his clothes every day "to gain my father's attention—he was a clothes hound." But his efforts failed, and their estrangement became complete during his late adolescence when Peter's father intuited that his son was gay. They did not reconcile until the last years of Mr. Sawyer's life, after he became a grandfather to Peter's brother's sons and stopped drinking. "Then," Peter said, "we could be real people to one another." Even though they continued to inhabit different worlds, father and son reached an unspoken understanding and some degree of mutual appreciation by the end, when Peter was able to comfort the dying man.

Then Peter's body, and his body image, metamorphosed. Freed from his father's judgments, when he had no more need to hide his identity or refute a truth that was no longer awful, he joined a gym. "I'd never gone to one before because he said only gays worked out there. I've felt stronger and much more real since I have." Demonstrating one of the most immutable (and unfair) differences between the sexes, Peter claimed, "My physique changed, and I lost weight without going on a diet—it was part of becoming myself and shedding who I had to be for him."

To his amazement, he found himself identifying after death with the man who never understood him while he was alive. "I liked my father's masculinity and started to seem more like him. I'm the patriarch of the family now." The changeling has stepped into his father's role literally as well as figuratively; he inherited some of his father's clothes and shoes, incorporated them into his wardrobe, and likes how he looks in them. When he shed who he had to be for his father, he embraced the paternal qualities that had real meaning for himself.

～～～

Physical pride and sexual satisfaction do not come easily to an incest survivor. A terrible chapter closes and a happier one opens when the mother who failed to protect her dies. "Two weeks after my mother's funeral I decided I wanted Larry, my current husband," said Alice Gerard. "I couldn't do it until then."

Alice described herself and her younger brother, who was also beaten and molested by their "bad seed" elder brother, as "raised by wolves—by parents who were utterly brilliant and utterly unequipped to have children." As her mother's favorite until she was "sold out" by her in adolescence, Alice held her mother particularly responsible because, unlike her father, she consistently denied the situation and never apologized.

When Alice's mother first became ill with the cancer that would kill her six years later, Alice, at age thirty, was going through the motions of a marriage. Her mother's illness prompted her to end the charade, and she decided to make showing dogs and participating in canine agility trials, the one physical connection she trusted, the center of her emotional life from then on.

Alice and Larry were friendly colleagues at the radio station where they were both producers; "I admired him although I never considered him appealing," she recalled. But something changed the night her mother died, and she found herself confiding in him. He came over to her apartment, comforting her with a tenderness that moved and terrified her; "I was so utterly laid bare in pain—I had to be in that state to let him touch me. I told him I'd been raped, about my mother, and that I never believed I'd live past age forty. He cried; he was afraid to hear it but he did, and he's been my ally ever since."

For the first time, she had found a man who was not damaged himself but who loved and honored her despite what she had been through, protecting her as neither parent ever had, offering something to live for. "There was nothing wrong with Larry. I couldn't believe there could be such a man, and such a family. Her death freed me to find him, and to love him."

It was critical to Alice that her mother had never met her beloved, "that he and she were completely separate." Only then could genuine physical intimacy be possible for her, without the taint of incest. "When she was alive, sex felt polluted; I could never make real love until she was dead. Then I could finally tell the truth. I stand so much taller." The conspiracy of silence and the fusion of sex with shame that were unavoidable while Alice's mother lived ended with her death. Alice held her head high—and walked into her ally's embrace.

Even a parent who is a real source of strength can have bad habits—and these bad habits can spur a surviving child into action. "My father was wonderful," said Maggie Brown. "He was always my protector, even when I was grown up—a powerful, very take-charge guy." He was also a heavy smoker, and Maggie, the child who was closest to him, was the only one of her siblings who shared his pack-a-day addiction. She identified with him as a smoker and also as a quitter. "I always thought I'd stop smoking when I was fifty-one, like he was when he did—that was my magic number," she recalled. But his sudden death warned her not to wait.

"I resolved to take charge and do it because I didn't want to die at seventy-eight like he did," she said. "His death accelerated the quitting process by three years—now's the time." Maggie had tried kicking the habit before, but on this occasion she went about it with the forethought and determination her late father had shown in other areas of his life. "I charted a plan. I took control of my life in a way I never had before; nobody else could do it for me. I knew that one of the things that kept me smoking was fear of gaining weight, so I decided to get disciplined. I gave myself eight to ten months after his death, and then that's exactly what I did; I joined a gym on February 1, a date I picked arbitrarily. That was ten years ago. I've never smoked since and never wanted to." Maggie turned her grief for her father and her identification with his best qualities into action on her own behalf; "It also gave me something positive to do other than just feel his loss."

Successfully stopping smoking right after her father died was the first of many efforts that increased Maggie's appreciation of her father's strength of character, and her own. "After his death I somehow came to admire him more, and in admiring him more I admired myself more because I'm like him. I'm fearless in the world because of him." She admires her model so much that she even appreciates the less-than-perfect physical traits she inherited from him. "See this extra fold of skin on my neck? It's not attractive, but I see my father when I look at it, because he had it, too. I look like him. He's part of me; I know he's with me. I don't walk alone." Now Maggie's father protects and encourages her from the inside.

⁓

Some parents inspire only by counterexample. The dissolution of their lives evokes shame, shock, and horror. Still, their children can profit if they can convert aversion into resolve to fight their own self-destructive tendencies.

Seeing the wreck her deeply depressed father had made of his life, his health, and his living space galvanized thirty-five-year-old Katie Lane to clean up her own act in every possible way. She was aghast by what greeted her when she opened the door to his apartment (her parents were divorced and she rarely saw her father) after his sudden death at sixty-three from a heart attack. Laid out before her were the ultimate consequences of the same self-neglect she was mired in herself; she recognized the warning and took it to heart. "It was the filthiest, dirtiest mess—so sad. I was a slob before I saw it, but now I clean like crazy."

Katie proceeded to address systematically everything her father had neglected. This involved changing habits she'd never thought about before. "I don't keep newspapers in the house because of all the newspapers I found piled everywhere—on the floor, on the table. I started to read the paper online so I don't have any type of paper lying around." Dealing with the smallest details of life can be psychic preparation for profound positive change.

Then she started paying attention to her body as well as to her environment. She became scrupulous about taking care of her health, the very thing he had neglected with disastrous consequences. "His sudden death was a wake-up call. His teeth were rotting—I have that vision in my head. When he was alive I didn't go to the dentist as much as I should have, so I started going regularly. I don't want to fall apart like him. I'm tackling my weight problem as well—I'm much more conscious of what I eat." Katie's brother also got the message and lost sixty pounds the year after their father died.

Father and daughter had been alienated for years (she described their relationship as "limited and detached") and were only beginning to reconcile when he died. "At the end of his life he was starting to show me affection—he'd given up on his own life," she said sorrowfully. But soon after cleaning out his apartment she had an experience that convinced her not to give up on hers. "I had an excruciatingly painful herniated disc and needed to see an orthopedist. I called my father's telephone number by accident and an orthopedist had taken over the number. It felt like my father was reaching out to me." Katie reconnected posthumously with the nurturing side of her father that had been so long buried. She was convinced that he was taking care of her at last.

Two years later, as reward for her efforts on her own behalf, Katie let her father help her in another way. "I used my inheritance to buy a beautiful co-op, and I got a cleaning lady. I made a vow to make a profound change. I saw his depression in me, saw it lurking, and I vowed to fight it. You think about how parents are supposed to be models—it's weird how they affect you after they die. I really didn't live my life before."

This thoughtful and courageous woman recognizes the profound significance of seemingly trivial, external changes. "I know many of the things I did are small things. I made these outward changes, little shifts in terms of cleanliness. They may seem superficial, but it's really a struggle with depression." It took six years for her to understand how her father's death made her a different person. "Interesting how you don't piece it together until a while after—I hadn't seen how his death affected me, but it did. I had to look at what he was and was not. Everybody carries their parents in themselves, of course; no matter what you do, you can't escape." But she was able to change the aspect of her father that defined her destiny, and as a happy consequence, "had more benefits from his death than when he was alive."

CHAPTER 6

TILL DEATH DO US PART

Marriage and Divorce

❧

Even in a society that abhors the notion of arranged marriages and supports a massive industry that dispenses advice on how to find Mr. or Ms. Right, our mothers and fathers "arrange" our mates for us far more often than we like to admit. Parents' personalities and their relationships with each other and with us provide the template for what we seek and what we avoid—which are frequently embodied in the same person. Science has shown that our spouses smell like our parents and resemble them in myriad other ways of which we are utterly unaware.

Years ago a dear friend and colleague introduced me to her fiancé, a man who looked so much like her father that anyone would have assumed they were father and son. When I mentioned this to her, she insisted that she had never seen the slightest resemblance—until she sat across the table from the two of them the next day and was shocked to see the same face on both the men in her life. The whole family got into the act; her brother, too, married a woman who was the spitting image of their mother and also had no clue that he had done so. In my friend's case the resemblance boded well, but often choosing somebody either like a parent, or whom a parent would like, is disastrous and cannot be undone until the person who inspired it need no longer be reckoned with.

Some parents have to die before their children can find a mate who truly suits them, or any mate at all; only then can they live a different life than their parents either exemplified or prescribed for them. This can eventually lead to marriages of true minds, to liberating divorces, and to many individually crafted permutations of partnerships that may suit the couple even if their parents would never approve.

⁓

My clever, curvaceous young friend Michelle Baker confessed to me that she had never been in love. I suspected as much because it had always seemed to me that her cats meant more to her (and treated her better) than her unsavory or unsuitable succession of boyfriends—the alcoholic Englishman, the autocratic fireman. I knew from the way she talked about her father when she was thirty-four years old that he was destined to be the only serious man in her life as long as he lived. Michelle thought so, too: "I knew that everybody I was with was wrong for me; they were placeholders," she admitted. Her father—domineering, difficult, but responsible—was always the one she turned to if she had a shelf that needed to be installed or an extra ticket to a football game. But his availability made her unavailable to anybody else. "If I ever needed him, he'd drop everything and be there," she said, "but I felt disloyal transferring my love to another man—slights hurt him deeply."

The only things Michelle's father failed to provide for his daughter were security and the right to a love all her own. His selfish demand for an exclusive attachment—inappropriate with a wife, let alone a daughter—caused him to interpret her natural needs as slights and transferrals of affection. Although she chafed under his constraints, she unquestioningly accepted his views and avoided conflict by never picking a man she could trust or respect. Infringements were punishable by fits of rage and severing contact, which had happened in her adolescence and which she had vowed never to endure again. She had long ago concluded that "if I do what I need to do to free myself and break away and find a relationship, I would push him away and maybe lose him altogether." Under the guise of taking care of her, he forced her to take care of him.

Like Jane Greenberg, whose flashy father took her on a weekend "date" to Paris when she was thirty-seven, Michelle functioned as a surrogate wife. She and her mother were rivals for life. "He had a lot more in common with me than with my mother—we were both social and shared interests like sports; I've always had more to talk about to him than to her," she said, with a sense of proprietorship that left no room for third parties.

Bristling at the suggestion that she might be lonely, Michelle presented herself as totally independent and never needing anybody. She seemed destined to spend weekends either at her parents' house, at bars seeking brief encounters, or at home with only feline companions for the foreseeable future. Then an ankle injury severe enough to require surgery gave her a chilling preview of what her life was likely to be if she continued on her present course. "It was a turning point—very depressing and very scary," she recalled. "My father insisted on taking me to the hospital at

5:00 AM, but he had gotten sick by then. I had to hail a cab and sit in the waiting room all by myself. I was so isolated; everybody else had someone with them. I'd never felt so alone. My father was the one I'd always turned to. He was no longer there. It was frightening—such a reality check. It reconfirmed everything I felt: this was not the life I wanted to live."

Michelle's father never recovered from his illness, and she took care of him devotedly until he died the next year. But after she lost him, she acted on her vow and answered an online ad. "I decided that I would absolutely make an effort; I wanted to find somebody. His death freed me of the obligation to put my father first."

The man she met when she put herself first was radically different from anybody she'd been interested in before—steadfast, opinionated, but not authoritarian. They were engaged within six months and married a year later. "I certainly see traits of my father in my husband. I could never be involved with a man like my father until he died," she told me. "I can turn things over to Charlie as I never could with anybody else—it would have been disloyal. I never felt the freedom to do it." At their wedding, I saw her joy when he looked lovingly down as she melted into his arms for their first dance. Love without loyalty tests could finally be hers.

Getting married was Michelle's way of disentangling herself from her father's demands after his death; getting unmarried may serve the same function. Most people consider divorce a monumental personal failure to be avoided at almost any cost. But for those who feel locked into an unsuitable marriage perpetuated at a parent's overt or covert behest, leaving is a personal achievement, an act of courage, and a source of pride.

It took thirty-seven years and his father's imminent demise for Dr. Daniel Weissman to leave a marriage he had long considered dead. "I'd felt imprisoned there for the last fifteen years, and it had to do with him," said this frank, thoughtful family practitioner. Daniel had been wretched and withdrawn for years but felt paralyzed because he was convinced that staying with a wife he no longer loved was the responsible thing to do, as his father had ordained. "He absolutely disapproved of divorce. He used to tell me, 'A man stays with his family.'" Daniel got the message that he would risk his reputation in his father's eyes, as well as his masculinity, if he left.

Even though Daniel was fifty-five years old, he couldn't bear to behave in a way his father deplored; the dangers of arousing paternal displeasure were too great and too familiar. Like Michelle, he accepted his father's definition of reality. Michelle's father had stopped talking to her when she displayed disloyalty by having boyfriends as a teenager, and Daniel's father was a "tough, scary character" who had punished his childhood rebelliousness by beating and rejecting him. While their fathers lived, freedom— for her to marry, for him to divorce—would have involved unsustainable losses.

But Daniel started to see things differently as his father's health deteriorated. Seizing this late opportunity, he spoke honestly to the elderly man, seeking his blessing and support— and got critical platitudes instead. "I went to see him and told him how unhappy I was, and all he could do was reiterate the old 'A-man-stays-with-his-family' line," Daniel said, with bitter sorrow that seven years had not erased. "I'd given him a last chance to be on my side and he failed."

Daniel also saw how his father had failed himself. "He was going downhill mentally and physically and had become very fixed in his ways. I was disgusted by what I saw—how unhappy, mean-spirited, and pigheaded he was. I saw his denial; he was having problems with incontinence and he wouldn't talk to the doctor; he tried to hide it. I thought to myself, 'This is ridiculous. I'm not going to play games with the truth like that. I don't want a life that replicates his; I'm not going to die living something inauthentic.'" His father's destructive masquerade mirrored his own bad faith.

Daniel had another epiphany around the same time. He went out of town for a conference, had a wonderful time, and came back deeply depressed. He had seen a female colleague he'd admired for years there and realized that he had fallen passionately in love with her. His depression when he returned home came from the torment of "knowing what I felt and wanted but not being able to act on it"—and he filed for divorce at long last.

Six days later his father was dead. "I couldn't live in a self-deluded state any more," Daniel declared. "I had to come out of hiding and get real with myself; I was giving advice to my patients and my children." His own sense of morality as a parent and a professional—as well as this intimation of his own mortality—demanded a different course of action than the one his father had practiced and preached. The father's death brought the son to life again before it was too late.

People typically justify continuing a troubled marriage for the sake of their children, but a more hidden motive, at least as compelling, is remaining for the sake of their parents. Daniel Weissman couldn't leave his wife for almost four decades because his father thought he should stay forever; Penny McDonald stayed with her husband for more than twenty years because her father thought she should never have married him in the first place.

Penny, a café owner in rural Massachusetts, was her father's favorite, but her position was tenuous because it was based on an impossible standard. "I was always trying to live up to his expectations, to what I thought he wanted; I struggled all my life to make him proud of me," she said. "His motto for me—not for the other siblings—was, 'Be your labor large or small, do it well or not at all,' so of course I turned into a compulsive perfectionist." The pressure was so great that the defiant perfectionist ran off at seventeen and married a man her father thoroughly disapproved of. Even though she soon saw the folly of her impulsive act (her husband turned out to be "distant and passive/aggressive"), she felt she had to stick out this very large labor and do it well to the bitter end. "I stayed with him for twenty-three-and-a-half years—because my dad told me it would never work," she admitted at age forty-six. "I'd fought him tooth and nail, and I had to defend my position. I felt I could never leave." Paradoxically, she wanted to make her father proud of her perseverance by proving him wrong; his precepts, rather than her own, ruled her life.

Penny's conversations with her father during his last illness changed her mind. "The shift in my thinking started as he was dying. I told him I'd spent my whole life trying to be perfect for him. He insisted he'd never expected that, but I pointed out specific instances when he had devalued my hard work. It gave me so much solace when he acknowledged that it was true, and apologized. It freed me, almost as if he gave me permission to leave. I went through changes—not physical ones, but thought changes, perspective changes." The most important change was that she got a divorce. "I used to think it would be a sign of failure to end my marriage," she said, "but the real failure was that I was staying for somebody else."

Few incentives to maintain a miserable marriage are as powerful as the need to prove a parent wrong—especially when it is coupled with an equally strong need to prove that you are different from that parent. For Aaron Goodman, whose father was famous not only as a psychiatrist but also as a four-times-married womanizer, staying in his own first marriage was imperative while his father was alive—even though his wife was unfaithful and he wanted out.

Since Aaron was two when his father divorced his mother, he was acutely conscious of the damage divorce wreaks. At fifty, he still dreaded repeating his father's behavior. "My pattern with women has been so similar to my father's. I want to leave every relationship—and I also choose women who can't be trusted. My father didn't like my wife; he always thought I should get out of the marriage, but I couldn't. My attachment to my wife and children was a weakness in his eyes." Even though Aaron accepted his father's judgment at face value, staying married was his way of demonstrating to the world that he was a more honorable, responsible husband and father than his own parent had been. Like Penny, he was so intent on contradicting his father's pronouncement that he could not know his own mind.

Aaron's head cleared when his father died. He saw that his marriage was a hopeless cause, and the couple parted. Visibly less tense and liberated from the compulsion to prove or to disprove anything, he proclaimed, "I feel much better."

                                  ✌

Mothers are as implicated as fathers in conflicts about divorce, although the dynamics differ. Adult children fear displeasing their fathers, and they fear devastating their mothers. Independent action becomes possible only when neither parent's responses must be taken into account.

For a discontented 1960s suburban housewife to find fulfillment in work and a more equitable second marriage is a familiar scenario—one that Sharon Black was unable to follow until she stopped justifying her mother's life by repeating it. Sharon had done everything her mother thought she should. She married a successful executive right after college, had children immediately, and settled uneasily into the role of the classic corporate wife. Since her husband's career required constant moves, she could never pursue a profession of her own but instead "managed to pick up interesting little jobs, like working on the local paper" wherever they went. Despite depression, headaches, and a sense of suffocation, she recalls "trying to live the life my mother wanted for me"—an airbrushed version of the one her mother wanted for herself.

The real reason why Sharon couldn't get a job was that she had an impossible one already. "I was always aware of my mother's vulnerabilities. She'd come from real poverty, married a wealthy man whom she was terrified of leaving, and never got an education. I learned very early that it was my responsibility to make things as nice for her as possible; I tried so hard to make her feel she was doing a good job."

Sharon's life changed dramatically when, at age thirty-five, she lost her mother to melanoma. "That permitted me to start to think more clearly about our relationship," she said. "I'd picked up her perspective, and I'd been afraid to live differently. In trying to please her I'd lived more traditionally than was comfortable for me." Sharon could see more clearly, and take action, when her mother was no longer in her line of vision. She divorced, went into therapy, went to graduate school, became a teacher of the disabled, and remarried in her forties. The despondency and the migraines disappeared. "I became much more open," she said, looking back with satisfaction at age sixty-five. "I discovered what I really wanted to do with my life; her death was enough of a trigger for me." No longer having to shield her mother from the painful facts of her own life precipitated Sharon's personal woman's liberation movement.

Carol Costas also had to protect her mother's equilibrium at her own expense. In her case, the sacrifice involved not daring to pursue a taboo relationship that would have recalled her mother's suffering, even if it meant losing a chance for happiness—until death made Carol's renunciation unnecessary.

Carol's father had a very public affair for eighteen years. It was all Carol knew of family life. "He had dinner with my mother and me every Saturday night, then got dressed and went out with his girlfriend," the thirty-seven-year-old lawyer recalled. "He treated my mother like dirt, so I was her ally. I used to see from her point of view only; I always thought that he was a bad guy and his girlfriend was a home-wrecking whore."

Naturally, Carol, who never married, felt like a traitor when she found herself intensely drawn to a married colleague in her firm. The distance she struggled to maintain quickly lost its enchantment when they began working on the same case. One day he confessed that he was only staying in his marriage out of guilt and told her that he planned to leave when his teenage daughter graduated from high school. The plot was familiar, but this time she herself was auditioning for the role of home wrecker.

Carol's mother was already ill with a brain tumor when the flirtation began. But not until she died six months later did her daughter go out to dinner with her colleague, where they finally held hands and declared their feelings openly. She behaved quite differently than any member of the original triangle had done. "I insisted that he make a decision. I told him I couldn't be a side salad or a mistress forever," she said with characteristic directness. "I needed a definite commitment that he was going to leave his wife if I was to keep seeing him, and I said that I wouldn't become sexually involved with him until he actually left her. I wanted a relationship in the open—my goal is a life. I must do this ethically. I won't lie and deceive."

There was no question in Carol's mind that she wouldn't have ever considered such a risky course before. "I would never have allowed us to explore something like this when my mother was around; it would have made her relive her pain and trauma. I would have spared her until it was a done deal. I wouldn't have let myself know I loved him. I had to wait until I didn't have to worry about how she would feel to know how I felt."

Carol's mother's death, in addition to permitting her to pursue a forbidden love, gave her a new perspective on her parents' marriage. "I used to see the situation exclusively from her side, but now I see more than just a woman scorned and a kid being hurt; I was too allied with my mother," she said. "I still believe the way my father and his girlfriend behaved was wrong, but seeing all sides dissipates my guilt." She no longer simply demonizes the lovers or idealizes her mother; Mrs. Costas looks less tragic and more selfish as a result.

Death helped Carol establish clearer boundaries between her mother and herself and revealed the uncomfortable truth. She figured out that her mother never wanted her to leave home or have a man of her own. "As a child I took care of her; she was depressed and I stayed home to keep her company. Later she was always trying to get between me and any man I wanted." Her mother's efforts were quite literal: every time Carol brought a boyfriend home and was about to kiss him, her mother managed to walk into the room. "She was always hindering my fun—particularly my sexual life, anything joyous with men."

Nothing but her own conscience hinders her now. Carol is acting like a responsible, dignified adult—one who knows her own mind and behaves better than either of her parents did in similar circumstances. When the time comes, the couple plans to marry and move to another state. "My mother would never have given my father an ultimatum like this. She needed to be a victim; I won't put up with disrespect. Something gave me the grace, faith, and patience to act as I have—things I never had before. I'm cleaning house." She is cleaning two houses, her parents' and her own. Death gave her the grace to do it.

తా

The death of Tom Campbell's father didn't inspire him to fall in love, or to end a bad marriage, or to begin living according to his own inclinations—it did all three. He emerged with a radically reconfigured identity. Two years later, this intense, self-aware forty-seven-year-old hospital administrator reported, "I've changed everything except my gender."

Tom could never do anything right, or be anything right, in his handsome, implacable father's eyes. Since childhood, he had lived with a pervasive sense of shame and failure. Tom described his father as "a man's man"—but one who felt compelled to compete with a boy. "My father found and created people to subjugate, people who were weaker," Tom said. "I had to be less physically able than he was, so I became grossly obese in high school. I made myself his inferior—inept, fat, and female," said this now-slender, soulful, and sophisticated man.

Tom sensed, but could not acknowledge at the time, that his father's hyper-masculinity and his need to denigrate his son came from doubts about his own sexual identity. "I understand now that he struggled with the same thing that I did, though he lived in a different world. He had a secret but developed internal life, and things leaked out. He told me once, 'You don't know what I went through.'" The covertly gay father rejected the son who embodied everything he hated in himself; their mutual shame sundered them.

Though Tom achieved national recognition and financial success in his field, the person he most needed to praise him never did. "I didn't let him in on the big moments because he would always disappoint me. I had money and power and a profession; he should have been prouder of my accomplishments," Tom said, still feeling the lack of his father's pride. The two were painfully estranged until days before his father died. The dying man asked Tom to be his health-care proxy, the only clear gesture of acknowledgment he ever made. The son, sadly in charge at the end, expertly carried out his father's wishes. Tom's father died on Tom's birthday.

He was a hard man to grieve for. "At the viewing of the casket, I could just kind of wave at him. Afterward I started bawling. So much wasn't said or dealt with—what a mess. We just missed always," Tom recalled, with real regret over their inability to connect.

Tom had married when he was thirty and had a daughter. Like his father, he continued to have a "secret but developed" inner world of homosexual fantasy, battling similar feelings of despair and self-alienation. But, unlike his father, he pursued psychotherapy for seven years and finally "accepted the bisexual, homoerotic part" of himself. He kept the knowledge private—although it, too, "leaked out." "I chose to live with it," Tom explained. "It was never a thing I was going to leave my marriage for; I felt I couldn't get out until one of us died." A death—his father's—did indeed provide the impetus for a long-overdue separation.

Tom remembered a conversation the two men had near the end that proved prescient. "I told him, 'I don't know what's going to happen, but nothing in my life will remain the same.' I didn't know exactly what that meant, but it was empowering as well as frightening. I'd always thought that everybody had to be a finished product by age twenty-five. My MO had been that I don't do change—and I've done nothing but change." He changed into a person who was no longer at war with himself.

Tom's forty-fifth birthday, his father's death-day, was the day his paralysis began to lift. He started questioning his assumption that his marriage was indissoluble. Now that the person he had always hidden from was gone, he found himself longing for a life and a love that he did not need to conceal from anybody. In his zeal for honesty, he decided to compensate for years of lying by telling the truth about his homosexuality to everyone important in his life. "I had to go around to people and bear witness that I'd made them collude, as if I were in a twelve-step program," he said—adding ironically that he got "all the distress and none of the pleasure" that such a disclosure might have brought to a more uninhibited sinner. In the next year, he and his wife separated. Later he made his first tentative steps toward having a relationship with a man who truly suited him, out in the open. "I'm able to live my life in a more authentic way," Tom told me. "This would not have happened had my father not died. I thought the wounds I carried would never heal, and in fact they're healing. It's like when something starts to itch—I feel itchy," he said with a laugh. "My father is my savior; his death blew out my repression like a fog. All of a sudden there is a clear blue sky."

❧

The critical element that both the newlywed and the too-long-married have in common was that their parents' voices—expressing expectations, needs, demands, prohibitions—were so pervasive that they were undetectable, yet so compelling that they drowned out every other sound. Their children could hear what they were saying to themselves, and act accordingly, only when these voices spoke no more.

CHAPTER 7

LIFTED UP IN MY MOTHER'S ARMS
Religious Epiphanies

༄

Religion binds us to our parents with unique, primordial power, just as it bound them to theirs. Even people who haven't set foot in a house of worship for years insist on having their children baptized or circumcised and feel the need to provide them with an education in the faith of their grandfathers and grandmothers—impulses that can wreak havoc in marriages between secular humanists of different backgrounds. Adults, including agnostic and non-practicing ones, give their parents a religious burial for the same reason: holding a wake or sitting shivah comforts survivors and reaffirms the continuity of a family's culture, providing ties to the past and links to the future.

The language of faith (God the Father, the Holy Mother) expresses the symbolic connection between Western religious belief and the parent/child relationship. Both God and parents create you, nurture you, and judge you; both are authorities to be obeyed. Perpetuating, reinterpreting, or repudiating a religious heritage after a parent's death has to be fraught with meaning.

Maintaining the family religious affiliation strengthens the bond with past generations. Children honor their parents' memories by making contributions to religious organizations or by becoming more active members of them; several men and women I interviewed mentioned how proud their parents would be that they were serving as presidents or on governing boards of their congregations. In the temple to which my family belonged, I recall three generations of sons in one family—who happened to be in the funeral business—blowing the shofar, the ritual ram's horn, on the High Holidays. I childishly thought it was a perk of the profession; in fact, the office had become unofficially hereditary.

Sometimes religion is the only sustaining connection to a parent that remains, as it was for Daniel Weissman, the physician whose father's pronouncement that "a man stays with his family" kept him unhappily married for decades. He rejected his father's unbending attitude toward divorce as a destructive falsehood but embraced his father's Judaism as truth, "the only tradition we still share." Attending services and running programs for his congregation keeps him in contact with the best in a deeply flawed deceased parent. A friend of mine who is an avowed atheist devotedly studies the Torah and attends an orthodox synagogue without any sense of cognitive dissonance for similar reasons; his only good childhood experience with his autocratic father was praying at his side.

Deciding which religious traditions to keep and which to discard is yet another aspect of "going through the stuff"; spiritual legacies are at least as charged as material ones. As a nonpracticing Reform Jew who has had no contact with organized religion since high school, I was surprised to find myself almost atavistically drawn to one particular ritual: the lighting of yahrzeit candles on the anniversary of a death, as I remember my mother doing to commemorate her parents. My father never lit them; his Jewish identity, like his parents', was strictly cultural, without faith or interest in observance. After the religious funeral I arranged for her, I was given the traditional candle that burns for the entire next week. I felt, with unexpectedly intense emotion, that the flame embodied her spirit, but kindling it seemed like part of the prescribed burial rite rather than an act of religious observance of my own. Two years later, however, I suddenly wanted to do what she had done. I bought the requisite twenty-four-hour candles that come in what look disconcertingly like water glasses with the kaddish, the ancient prayer for the dead, printed on their labels (since I live in New York City, the supermarket in my apartment building had a supply), and I lit them not only for my parents but also for my analyst who died suddenly thirty years ago and for my husband's mother—neither of whom were Jewish. In this way I, who chose to have no children myself, took my place among the generations of mourners.

A patient of mine who was raised in a strict orthodox household had a more conflicted and complicated ritual-sorting task than mine; she still identified herself as a believer, and traditional religions don't exactly sanction the have-it-your-way approach. She had recently joined an amateur chorus and was enjoying singing in concerts with them on weekends. But what was she to do when rehearsals were held on Saturdays? Both her parents were dead, and her devout siblings lived in distant cities, so it was now legitimate for her to pursue a don't ask/don't tell policy about Sabbath observance—particularly since she hadn't followed it to the letter for years in her own home. She frankly admitted that not having to worry about wounding or offending her parents was a relief. Their absence not only permitted her to do things she had never done before but also to think independently about which aspects of her heritage she wanted to retain because they were still personally meaningful and which to reject because they had become rote. These were questions and choices she could not have even formulated without committing sacrilege while they were alive.

Similarly, some people only feel free to marry outside their faith when they are orphans, breaking a taboo essential to their parents but irrelevant to themselves. Following one's own religious convictions after a parent dies—or rejecting religion altogether—no longer has shock value and is therefore more likely to be a seriously considered decision rather than merely a rebellion.

Converting to another religion is a radical departure from one's spiritual "home." Those who do so are not simply reinterpreting or moving away from what their parents practiced. They are, literally, turning into something else by joining another "family" of the faithful. The convert exchanges one identity for another; being "born again" of necessity symbolically rejects those responsible for your birth the first time around. Many people cannot take this step while their parents are alive, either because they wish to avoid causing pain or fear provoking outrage. But because a belief system of some kind is an integral part of most families, relationships with deceased parents always play a role whenever children embrace, lose, change, or reconceive their spiritual identities.

❧

Converting to a faith different from the one you were born into can reflect a need to punish parents, to separate from them, or even to recover them. Posthumously severing a tie with a difficult parent by adopting a new religion paradoxically expresses the very connection the convert flees—particularly if he embraces that faith with a vengeance. Ben Marks's mother was, according to her right-wing son, a "hard-nosed atheist"; worse, she was a "born-again Democrat"—as well as "one of the most self-righteous people you'd ever meet," a trait her son shares more than he realizes. The intensity of his scorn ten years after her death suggests how combative their relationship was, but more complicated feelings underlay it; he still misses her. "I'm surprised at how painful her death is," Ben admitted. "We used to be best friends. I was closer to her than to anyone else in the family until I got married." Although he attributes their estrangement to his mother's jealousy of his wife's superior housekeeping talents, more basic rivalry was to blame.

Seven years after her death, Ben committed an even graver act of betrayal by becoming a Catholic. "I felt I'd be at home there," he explained, seeking a sense of comfort unavailable in his original one. He never would have risked it before. "She would have found it absurd—if you're intelligent you just don't do such a thing. I'd have faced withering hostility, even if she'd have been nice about it. I always wanted to please my mother; the idea of her not liking you as she once did or having less respect is pretty painful," he said, using the present tense to describe judgments he still fears. Having lost her respect for one life choice, he couldn't do it a second time.

Ben's motives for converting were complicated, even contradictory. He was rejecting a mother who rejected him and also asserting himself in a way he found impossible while they lived together. "When I didn't have to worry about her criticism any longer I could look at things purely from my own point of view," he said.

"I've always loved the truth; I never would have made as much progress in getting to know it with her around—she was such an inhibiter." Still, he remembers her as "very loveable and funny" and describes himself as someone who "always questions dogma." Even though he claims that "as I became more religious I didn't miss her at all," he continues to be involved with her. The man who questions dogma also accepts with equanimity (and disguised pleasure) that his mother is "going to hell because she isn't saved." It may be a source of unconscious comfort that, if he is indeed heaven-bound himself, her fate would free him of her influence for all eternity. He leavens this judgment—one far harsher than any of hers—by "believing in a God of infinite second chances." He has found Someone more forgiving than either the mother or the son, Who may still arrange a final rapprochement between them.

A new religious identity offers peace and purpose, the comfort of community, a haven from a traumatic history and from parents who failed. It is a way to save yourself emotionally as well as spiritually. Pam Kaplan transformed herself from an upper-middle-class "gourmet Jew" into a working-class, born-again evangelical Christian to regrow roots that were tragically torn away. The death of her father was a prerequisite.

When Pam was a teenager, her parents violated every principle of Jewish family life and the sanctity of the home. Her mother had an affair with her father's business partner, who also happened to be his brother. After a punishing divorce, she married her lover/brother-in-law and had what Pam described as a "nightmare marriage." Meanwhile, her father ran off with a woman he'd known for six weeks and "shed his whole family"—including Pam, who never ceased longing for him. "I was numb because I'd grown up in a big Jewish family," she explained. "One of my most painful memories was being in graduate school and not being invited anywhere for the holidays; nobody knew what to do with us. That was the point at which I cut loose—I stopped being a nice Jewish girl." The lost and desperate young woman rejected the religion whose members, both inside and outside her family, abandoned her.

Pam, who had once been "groomed for life as a Jewish-American Princess," needed to radically redefine her identity in order to reclaim it. The East Coast sophisticate whose religious experience was superficial moved to Colorado, where she found fulfillment working as a waitress and a janitor. ("I'd never touched the ground growing up," she said.) Her Christian neighbors reached out to her as her original coreligionists never did and introduced her to what became her true faith—one as far removed as she could imagine from her own family's. "They had a purity of life that was nothing like mine," Pam recalled. "Through them I met a man—which I can only ascribe to the spirit of God. I told him how unhappy I was. He asked me, 'Will you consider having Jesus save your life?' I was so lost that I was open to Him." Thirty-five years later, she is still open.

Pam attributes her salvation in part to her father's death; as authentic as her adopted faith feels, she knows she would have needed to spare him from it. "Even though he walked away from me, I still care so much about his good opinion that if he had lived and we'd had a relationship again I'd never have done this to him. Nothing could dislodge the fact that I adored him. He taught me how to drive, and I had patience and ease when I taught my son as a result. He was reassuring, and his love was always there." Her love for her father—based on genuine tenderness and encouragement before their break—has never died, as Pam's recent dream confirmed:

> I dreamt that my father was walking down the hall from my son's bedroom and had his arm around him. I said, "Daddy, where have you been?" He was so real that I woke up weeping; there was something of eternity about it, something in our connection that is eternal.

God the Father has not replaced her father; her experience of divine paternal love is a natural, undying extension and transformation of what she never fully lost.

Memories of mothers and fathers can provide religious inspiration after they are gone, and many children attribute their renewed faith to a parent's posthumous presence in their lives. Since everybody feels like a little child again in a crisis, the parent who sustained you best shapes your image of divinity. It is natural for God to assume a maternal aspect for a man who turned to his mother for consolation; even the most traditional dogma can have a uniquely personal manifestation that reflects the parent/child relationship at its core.

I never thought of my acquaintance Joe Bailey, a fifty-three-year-old philosophy professor with bright eyes and a darkly sardonic manner, as a religious person, much less a mystic. This wiry, worldly scholar, brimming with contained energy, does not suffer fools gladly and seems far too realistic—even cynical—for visions. Yet the dream he told me that reconnected him to his childhood faith through the intercession of his dead mother would do any saint proud.

Like many intellectuals, Joe had left his naïve and devout past—he'd been an altar boy—far behind. The ardent piety of his youth didn't jive with his fast-paced professional life as he climbed the academic ladder, where the competition is more bloodthirsty than in any corporation because the universe is smaller, and publish-or-perish is the norm. "I'd been very religious into high school," Joe told me, "but I became a too-smart-to-be-Catholic kind of guy, so nonpracticing and so aggressively secular." Even as he became irreligious, he continued to adore and identify with his "funny, fabulous" mother, who died when he was forty-one. She, too, did everything with passion; Joe remembers her falling to her knees in prayer every night when he was a child. Until he wrote her eulogy, however, he didn't realize the full power of her belief, nor its continuing hold on him. "My mother was heroic emotionally, larger than life. Her brother was an alcoholic suicide, and her sister died of cancer. She was the sole survivor of her family, but she never carried that baggage around at all. What an example of how to respond to consummate losses! I could only take full account of her achievement when she died." Catholicism and character got her through, he realized, and after her death he began to relate to her spiritually as well as emotionally. "My resonance with spirituality stirred up again very intensely. I felt an acute need for the church—a deep reaction, deeper than habit." Despite the life he led, the bereaved son's renewed hunger for faith reflected his primal connection to his profoundly religious mother.

In stages, as he assumed more roles in adult life that mirrored his mother's, the devout secularist returned to the fold. When Joe married a year after her death, he was "adamant" about a church wedding, even though it required his wife to go through the arduous process of obtaining an annulment from her first, non-Catholic, husband. His religious fervor grew after their daughter, who was named for his mother, was born the following year. The

Catholicism of his childhood was by then reestablished as a living part of him, without apology—but not without conflict. "Of course I had to wrestle with my rational side," Joe conceded, "but I was having a real experience of faith that was much more than looking back into a set creed or series of habits."

Then, during the worst crisis of his life, Joe's experience of faith took a quantum leap into mystical ecstasy. The first two years after his daughter's birth were miserable; Joe and his wife were fighting all the time over everything ("finances, work, travel commitments, daily schedules") as they tried to manage two demanding careers, two strong egos, and parenthood. Divorce was out of the question, and happiness seemed illusory. "Marriage was feeling like combat, and every day was enormously stressful," he said, recalling the tension that had torn him apart. The nonrational side of him, his mother's legacy, came to his aid; in his darkest moment, Joe "all of a sudden" had a dream of "real and personal deliverance":

> I was simultaneously observing and in the dream. I was an infant baby in a crib and I was distressed, crying and wailing. I felt an unbelievable sense of comfort when a pair of arms—my mother's, but disembodied—reached down and picked me up. The feeling of being lifted was tangible: relief from stress, symbolic affirmation. There was a sense of otherness, of spiritual life. It almost felt like ancestor worship.

Joe's dream depicts an extraordinary psychological and spiritual journey. His rapturous contact and consolation felt both subjective and objective, personal and universal. The repetitive term "infant baby"—striking in so articulate a man—shows how anguish made him inarticulate as he wept, helpless and alone, like an abandoned infant. The arms that reached down to lift and cradle him (and which he believed would eventually raise him to heaven and to reunion) were "disembodied" because they represented the arms of his actual, now-dead mother, merged with an image of God, Who has no body. For Joe, God is a mother. "This dream has never gone way. It's continued to console me," he said, with mingled intensity and calm. Ten years later, her arms have not let him down.

The "light" that "went back on in terms of religious life" for Joe Bailey illuminates many adults whose parents have died. Some it leads back as a living memorial to the rituals their parents performed; some it leads away to other, nonfaith-based sources of truth that replace their parents' beliefs—and some it leads beyond, to another state of consciousness altogether, one that incorporates and transcends the deepest love they knew.

CHAPTER 8

A Voice of My Own

Creative Self-Expression

⁓

After my mother died, I had to write about it. I knew I was going to do so well in advance. This was not the first time she would inhabit a book of mine—our relationship has appeared in every one—but this time there was a difference: I had a premonition that something was going to change radically in my life as a result of her death, though I had no idea what it would be; the conviction was based on blind faith. But I had no doubt that I would discover this change, comprehend it, articulate it—and maybe even bring it about—by documenting it. The grieving/integration process and the creative process were intermingled for me.

Dead parents live again in memoirs, plays, and poems by writers like Colette, Eugene O'Neill, and Sylvia Plath. Writing—as well as other artistic pursuits like painting, composing, singing, dancing, or acting—are concrete ways to celebrate beloved memories or to resolve tormenting ones. Artists conjure their parents in their work to bring them back, to lay them to rest, or to say aloud what could never be said to them in person. Some people produce their best work after they are orphaned, and others cannot produce any work at all until then because they cannot contact their deepest selves in a parent's presence. In either case, the living parent is an inhibiting—or even paralyzing—force. Parental loss also has a positive impact on the expressive life of people who are not professional artists, freeing them to discover their own viewpoints and to find their medium.

～

A friend of mine gave a dramatized reading of her poetry that I attended. One of the works she presented was a lament addressed to her mother's corpse, its classic meter and formal structure containing the passionate anguish it expressed. The bereft daughter gazed once again at her mother's painfully pinching earrings and constricting outfit as she lay in her coffin, sorrowing that even there she could not relax. The audience quietly wept, in solidarity and identification. "For some people the state of orphanhood is terrifyingly lonely and for others, like me, it brings great solitude; they leave space for you," she told me afterward when I congratulated her, my eyes still wet with tears. Although she had published many volumes of poems and given readings for years, this was her first staged performance—an artistic step she could not take before.

Another friend of mine, also a poet, spoke in verse to her dead mother about how she had emotionally starved both of them. In the last line, flat and plain because the feeling had been wrung out of it, she said that she had never been able to connect with this woman, who was paradoxically no more inaccessible or insubstantial in her grave than she had ever been. The line was repeated like an incantation—as much to force herself to face this wretched truth as to tell the reader what her mother could never hear. Writing this poem inspired her to take the ultimate communication risk herself; she left her job as a copy editor at a publishing house ("that was the way I could stay hidden," she admitted) to concentrate on writing poetry full-time. No longer a midwife for the self-expression of others, she chose to speak directly to an audience with the capacity to listen. "I was always afraid my ideas in verse weren't good enough," she said. "Now I don't care; they're mine."

Patients of mine who are not published writers also found themselves inspired to produce poems, essays, short stories—even blogs and diary entries—to express and work through the experience of losing their parents—as well as a host of ideas unrelated to their parents.

Putting words on paper is an effective way to work through a parent's death—particularly one who is difficult to mourn. Alice Gerard, the radio producer "raised by wolves" who discovered sexual pleasure only after she lost her mother, published an essay about helping her beloved dog die; it permitted her to grieve by proxy.

Alice's twin passions were freelance writing and competing in canine agility trials with her shrewd and sprightly Border collie Zoe. Before she met her current husband, her bond with animals had been the most enduring and satisfying thing in her life. It was also a connection she shared with her troubled mother, who had failed to intervene when Alice's brother molested her. "She had thirteen animals. It's completely understandable that some of us can love them better than we can love people," Alice remarked.

Alice's sister was scandalized that she decided to compete in a race when their mother was failing. "She couldn't understand that I had to do it in order to get myself to the funeral." Zoe's companionship helped her feel grounded enough to visit her mother at the end and to try to reconcile. "I knew she was dying and I hated her and I knew that wasn't where I wanted to end up. When I went to see her, I was able to say, 'I love you—you know that, don't you?' I was feeling desperate to hear it back, but of course she couldn't do it, so I did it by myself in therapy." Art was her way of grieving.

A tragic but timely opportunity to help a dying creature, one she loved unambivalently, presented itself soon afterward. Zoe was horribly injured in an accident and had to be euthanized. Alice elected to hold her and comfort her, looking into her eyes and communicating wordlessly, to the end. "It was my privilege to do so," she said in an essay about Zoe and the parallel with her mother's death that was published in a literary magazine later that year. "It was the best thing I've ever written," she said. "When I'm with the dogs I love I'm with her. After her death, by writing about my grief, we could see each other."

Singers communicate in their own voices even more directly than writers do. For that reason music provides a natural outlet for those whose self-expression was stifled by a parent's oppressive presence. A patient of mine signed up for voice lessons soon after her mother's funeral. "Since she criticized whatever I said, I had to silence myself in order to be with her," she told me. "I held my breath for fifty years, never knowing what I wanted, was good at, or enjoyed. I'm learning to sing because I need to hear my own voice; that's the only thing I want to do. It's amazing that I've discovered this now."

Cindy Atkins, the teacher who moved her mother's furniture en masse into her apartment and was afraid to wear the diamond ring she had inherited, allowed herself to join an a cappella choral group five years after she was orphaned. "My mother's marriage was the end of her playing the piano," Cindy said. "I'd always wanted to sing, but I didn't ever think about actually doing it until lately. I couldn't sight-read and I figured I'd have to learn, but I finally decided to try anyway and it's been fantastic. Singing has brought me closer to her." A love of music was one of the few positive things that the mother and daughter had in common; becoming a performer in her own right despite obstacles was Cindy's way to take possession of something her mother had relinquished. She sang for them both.

❧

Art is the ultimate form of self-expression. Certain people with artistic talent are so engulfed by their relationships with parents who are depressed, self-involved, or domineering that they are unable to plumb their own depths. Negotiating these daunting relationships leaves little energy for inner exploration. When such a parent dies, it is as though a hidden reservoir gushes forth; no one inhibits the flow any longer.

Death made a novelist out of Dennis Morrison. The need to express everything he didn't get to say to his father on his deathbed galvanized him to re-create the scene as it should have been in his first work of fiction. After thirty-two demoralizing years as a teacher of English as a second language, Dennis found his true calling to tell his own story. In the process he not only worked through the painful residue of their relationship but found what had eluded him his whole life: a source of pride and purpose that astonished him.

I knew Dennis in high school. He was one of those awkward, unhappy, bespectacled smart kids who is uncomfortable in his own skin. Until we spoke forty years later—he had written me when my first book was published and later he sent me his first— I had no idea of the shame and torment he was subjected to during his teenage years by his father, a beaten-down insurance agent. "My father was always jealous of me and my mother's affection for me, and he took it out on me by what he called 'teasing,' but it was really abuse," he told me. "I used to dread when he was in the house—I was a sensitive kid, and he'd humiliate me and reduce me to tears. He still had this effect on me when I was nineteen years old." Dennis hated his father with barely suppressed violence, his helpless rage breeding dreams of vengeance. "I came within a hair's breath of slugging him. I had fantasies of his dying as a punishment for what he was doing to me," he admitted, as if confessing a crime.

Things changed radically for the better after a stroke forced Dennis's father to retire. "He very gradually began to mellow. The tantrums stopped. I started to serve a useful function by taking care of my parents' house when they went away. He and I became friends; it was a gift from God."

By the time Mr. Morrison had a major heart attack ten years later, he and his son had become genuinely intimate. "As he declined we got closer and closer. I read him a story right before his operation. I was his driver, and I went to see him every night. He suffered dreadfully in that last year, but he never lost his dignity, gentleness, or sense of humor. He became almost saintly; I never suspected that would be possible. I truly loved him," Dennis said, tenderness and anguish replacing the ferocity in his voice.

But as his father's condition worsened and death approached, Dennis was horrified to find his own ill feelings resurfacing. Unconsciously fearing that his old deathwish had come true, he was seized with the compulsion to confess:

It all came back to me, and I was filled with despair. I felt terrible guilt when I saw that he was dying—which is what I had wanted. He'd been purified by his suffering, but I hadn't been redeemed by anything comparable; I was healthy, and I was alive. I had an overpowering need to try to tell him how monstrous I felt that I'd hated him then and loved him now. We were both at fault. I knew it was my last chance, so I sat by his bed and tried to do it, but he stopped me. He brushed it aside and said, "We understand each other, son." He wouldn't talk about the deepest feelings; he didn't want to hear the words, so I ended up saying it to myself. But something was incomplete.

Saying it to himself was not enough to expiate his intolerable guilt. Like Alice Gerard, Dennis had to tell everyone what his parent could not hear. The "incomplete" scene was completed in a redemptive novel, which he used his inheritance to publish. The hero bears the author's nickname, and the tale—funny, sad, and deeply touching—is told by his sharp-witted, perceptive little niece. At the end of the book he recounts to her the climactic deathbed scene of mutual forgiveness between himself and his estranged father; she is the one who "writes" it down and tells the world in his behalf. The reviews were good—a feat almost unheard-of for a self-published first novel. "I tried to find a way—a devious and unusual way—of expressing my grief and pain at my feelings about my father," the author explained. "I had that story take place offstage because I couldn't bear to be too explicit—I still couldn't say those things directly." Even ten years after the fact, the scene is still too hot for him to handle. The reconciliation and self-forgiveness he craves may take more time—and another book—to achieve.

The poetically fractured language Dennis employs ("self of steam" for "self-esteem," for example) is based on his students' misspellings over the years—mistakes that had convinced him his life's work was as pointless and humiliating as his father's, but that he now transmuted into a source of pithy, merry wordplay. From these unlikely materials, he fashioned his own brand of English as a third language. "It all came from a part of me that's not really conscious," he said. "I couldn't have thought this up. I'm not really that smart, but that part of me is a genius. I used so much of myself; it amazes me that I was able to do it, to grasp my personality so fully. I created a work of fiction with no background. It really took incredible nerve—that's such a strong thing for my identity. I'm so thrilled with it, so totally delighted that I did it. I happen to love my little book. It has my heart and soul. Instead of my life having been a failure, now it's a success."

≈∽≈

In common parlance, "to act" means to pretend, to fake it, to hide behind a mask. But for Beth Grant, it means just the opposite: committing herself to study acting seriously at age forty-nine after her parents died was throwing away the mask and revealing her authentic self to the world.

There was something smart and spirited about Beth—she is the high school teacher who so thoughtfully integrated her mother's belongings into her apartment and redesigned the diamond ring she inherited to suit her own taste—but she hid her own sparkle behind a muted, matronly façade. Never married, she dedicated her life to her students and to reluctantly doing the bidding of her angry, histrionic, critical, and endlessly needy mother, the only one in her traditional Catholic family with a license to show emotion. Her father, less overtly demanding, was cut off and committed to keeping the peace; her sister led a constricted, conventional life as a wife and mother. As a young teenager, Beth liked to sing and dance but never pursued either; she was so nervous when she tried out for the church choir that her throat closed up and no sound escaped. She was the last person you would ever imagine who could come to blazing life onstage.

Despite her ambivalence and her feeling that the world was passing her by, Beth spent her forties as a caretaker, nursing first her father, then her mother, until their deaths. Then she realized how much her relationship with her parents had consumed and structured her existence; without them and with no family of her own, what was she going to do with her time? Searching through catalogs for classes to take, an all-day improvisation workshop for beginning actors caught her eye. She held her breath, quelled her fears ("Will they think I'm ridiculous or pathetic?" she wondered), and signed up.

She got hooked immediately. To her amazement, the woman who had played no role but dutiful daughter in her parents' house felt entirely at home playing all kinds of women (including one very like her own mother) onstage. There, being free, frank, and expressive came naturally; what she had had to conceal for years she was suddenly encouraged to show.

The experience was a revelation. "Immediately I knew: acting is the real me," she exclaimed. What she discovered on her first day intensified with each new class she took. She loved exploring the characters she portrayed; interacting with the other actors; and most of all, taking in the response of the audience, which she found as "energizing" as her original maternal audience had been enervating. With every performance, the woman who had always acted smaller than life felt herself grow larger. "How foreign and how comfortable this is at the same time," she reflected. "It's incredibly exciting to find myself in such an alien environment, one that I never imagined being part of. How can I explain this to people? Acting shifts the whole world—living differently, thinking differently—this huge, exciting world is so remote from my family; it's like turning on a light in a room."

The theater was a brightly illuminated room all her own where, at last, the spotlight was on her. "My mother took up all the emotional space, so I had to fit into what was left over," Beth explained. "As her daughter I always had to be self-deprecating, always on the sidelines. This is my first opportunity to be the center of attention, a second chance at something I didn't get right the first time: self-expression. I want to do it for the rest of my life." At an age when most aspiring actresses have either made it or given up, the acting bug bit her hard.

Fortunately, she also discovered that she had talent.

Over the next two years, Beth enrolled in a professional acting school, had headshots made, and with the encouragement of her teachers went on her first professional auditions. After she won her first role, in an educational film, the director noted that she had "a nice natural quality, vulnerability, and effervescence." Her ambition is realistic: she wants to pursue acting full-time after she retires from the school system in five years—and she'd love the occasional paying gig in character parts or voice-overs.

Beth knows that finding her vocation (and the financial means to pursue it) was made possible by the deaths of her parents. "Acting comes from a part of me that my parents never knew or would have approved of; it's so out there. Only now can I be visible and audible; I could never expand in their presence. I could never have done any of this while they lived."

One of the things acting gives her is the right to make mistakes. She invited friends to attend a performance, something she had never done in her life. "It's a real triumph for me to allow people I know to watch me. I'm no longer constantly worried that I might do something wrong, as I always was around my mother," she said. "I used to be afraid to open my mouth, afraid to say something stupid—but in acting, making mistakes is part of the process. I am more myself in a very public way, the opposite of what my life had been. I'm out there saying, 'This is who I am.' I can be on stage without hiding. I never could have gotten here if she was still on this planet—I couldn't think straight. I couldn't take these risks with her breathing down my neck."

Since Beth also loves her mother, she envisions her as an appreciative audience in the hereafter. "I have a sense of her supporting me now. I hope there's an afterlife so she's looking down and feeling happy for me; she wanted me to blossom but didn't realize she was blocking it. I was attached to both my parents, but I could not live as long as they were living. There was never enough air for me to breathe without my feeling like I was stealing it from them. Acting turned out to be the perfect antidote to my childhood."

Like other parent-haunted artists, amateur and professional, Beth has taken her place at center stage. But her mother and her father had to make their final exits before she could do it.

PART III

ORPHANS' BENEFITS

Seeing Parents with New Eyes

CHAPTER 9

FATHER KNOWS BEST?

The Punitive Parent Dies

꧁꧂

A huge ash came crashing down three years ago in the woods by my house in upstate New York, toppling saplings and even large trees in its wake. It was painful to see the fallen giant lying helplessly horizontal, paradoxically a more commanding presence in its demise than when its girth was hidden by masses of foliage. The green moss and grey lichen encrusting it up to its crown, the herringbone pattern of its bark—and, within its sheared-off trunk, evidence of the disease that had caused its death—were all exposed. This spring, though, I noticed something unexpected: in the clearing created by its fall, a grove of red trilliums, my favorite wildflower, had sprung up, their deeply veined leaves unusually large and opulent and their maroon flowers more fleshy than any others in the vicinity. Young plants long unable to flourish under the living ash's shadow now had light and air and room to grow.

Dictatorial, oversized parents have a similar suppressive effect on their children's aspirations. Families revolve around them.

Their sons and daughters spend inordinate amounts of time longing for their blessing, quaking at the possibility of their displeasure, striving desperately to satisfy their demands or meet their expectations—and almost always falling short.

I remember an old friend of mine, a brilliant student, recounting with shame years after the fact that her college career had been a sore disappointment to her father. Even though she had graduated summa cum laude and Phi Beta Kappa from Harvard, she was not, he made sure to remind her, class valedictorian. Knowing rationally that his reaction was preposterous—he would have found something else to criticize even if she had achieved that honor too—did not keep her from blaming herself and feeling like a failure. Even though she has never shed his impossibly high standards entirely, my gifted friend was one of the fortunate ones who did eventually figure out how to create her own destiny while her father was still alive. Many others discover themselves only when, like my ash, the colossus topples.

Unpleasable parents come in both genders (though she was herself a chef, Diane Gordon dared not cook in her omnipotent mother's kitchen), but tyranny is more typical of fathers; mothers are more likely to express their own bottomless demands via depression and accusations of neglect. In either case, insecurity, competitiveness, dissatisfaction with their own lives, or the compulsion to reenact their negative experiences with their own parents (with the roles reversed) prevent them from feeling unalloyed pride or joy. Sadly, even children who admire such parents breathe a sigh of relief when the pressure is off.

Sherry Taylor's therapist suggested that she contact me because of the remarkable change that came over her after her father died; she had practically sprouted wings. "He was controlling, critical, and negative about everything I did," said the sprightly forty-five-year-old administrative assistant, "and it affected me terribly. I was so depressed and fearful that I couldn't make a decision about anything—even buying a lampshade—without agonizing over whether people would like it. The only thing that mattered to me was doing the right thing, and pleasing my father." Fortunately, her excruciating indecision and hypervigilance propelled her to seek help while he was still alive.

When Mr. Taylor finally died at age eighty-four—as a matter of course Sherry had moved him into her house and tried unsuccessfully to meet his demands until his final hour—a miraculous change came over her. "I became a different person," she said matter-of-factly. The woman who couldn't select a lampshade without having an anxiety attack served shrewdly and confidently as executor of her father's estate. Nobody was more surprised than she. "I dealt with everything—money, plans, the house. At first all I did was worry about what everybody else in my family felt, and needing to be fair. Then one day I opened my eyes and said, 'Fair? Things were never fair'—and gave myself a few extra bucks without feeling bad about it. I told my siblings that I had done more and I deserved more, and nothing disastrous happened." When she started thinking for herself, she discovered that she had a knack for it; she became her own authority. Nobody would ever again have the power over her that her father once wielded.

Sherry's self-confidence kept growing. "I've continued to get better—more capable of doing things and living my life," she said. "Little everyday things still amaze me." One not-so-little thing she did last year was to plan and book a vacation without relying on—or even consulting—anybody else. "When I told my family what I'd done, I could almost hear them thinking, 'Who *are* you? And what have you done with our mother?'"

Timorous no longer, she turned out to be as competent a parent as she was an executor and a travel agent. "I used to be in a panic about raising my children, but now I think things through. My relationship with my father affects me as a mother—every day I try to say something positive to them. I'm a lot more independent, and my husband's very happy about it."

Sherry's demeaning father was neither an obvious brute nor a drunk, and he was closer to her (she was the baby of the family) than to his other children, but his relentless negativity unleavened by tenderness had the same effect as cruelty. Now no one punishes her for being herself any longer. Although not oblivious to the needs of others, she pays attention to her own. "When I was a child, my father noticed everything I did, always waiting for a mistake. I don't feel like I'm being watched all the time anymore. It didn't happen overnight, but it's gone now. I really don't care what anybody thinks," she exclaimed with a delighted laugh. "I've been freed from prison."

There are many ways to make offspring feel inadequate. Some parents, like Sherry's father, do it by constantly criticizing and actively undermining. Others, like my friend's father, make it clear that nothing you do is ever good enough. A more subtle but equally effective technique is to become—as my own mother did—The World's Foremost Authority, whose heights no child can ever reach. These daunting but secretly insecure figures need to demonstrate their superiority to the very children from whom they expect the most; why else would a grown man or woman compete with a child?

The father of an acquaintance of mine was an accomplished jazz saxophonist who gave up a promising career to become a hearing-aid salesman. Though he encouraged his son's considerable talent on the same instrument up to a point, trouble started when the son turned professional. Every time he started practicing—he lived at home in his early twenties—his father would mysteriously begin playing along in another room, just loud enough to throw him off and make him feel shrill and awkward. Despite his own successful career, he remained convinced that his father was the superior musician.

Though few children of secretly or openly competitive parents escape unscathed, those of the same sex—especially sons of overbearing fathers—suffer most. They often have to wait until their idols and their jailers die to discover themselves.

Michael Meredith was a towering, if remote, presence in the lives of his three children. A man of strong opinions with no scruples about expressing them, he had built an impressive real estate empire, served on the boards of many charities and arts organizations, and managed to make everybody around him feel simultaneously awestruck and incompetent. His imperial manner undermined the confidence of both his daughters ("He'd always point out your weaknesses," the younger one told me), but Ken, his eldest child and only son, bore the brunt.

Ken Meredith was not the son his father wanted. Artistic and musical since boyhood, he was always "nontraditional, definitely not the corporate type." Since childhood Ken felt that being a jazz drummer was his real vocation, but he knew that his "very strict, classic authoritarian" father, with whom he had been locked in combat for as long as he could remember, would be furious. "We both had strong personalities. My earliest memory was my father aggressively opposing everything that interested me; in his perfect world I would have been into sports and collecting baseball cards. He thought my music was subversive and a bad influence on me, though I never understood why." Mr. Meredith required his male heir to be a carbon copy, and the only way his son could assert himself was to sabotage everything his father expected of him.

Not surprisingly, college was a disaster. "I wasn't ready, but he expected me to be on a path of fame and glory. I was just not into it. I never showed up for class. I completely blew it off, and eventually dropped out. I wasted my parents' money and felt terrible about it." Things spiraled downward as Ken, now nineteen and a failure in both his own and his father's eyes, dropped out of college a second time, got kicked out of the house, and sank into depression.

Since he had to pay his rent, he turned to his favorite uncle, a real estate lawyer, who gave him a job as a paralegal in his firm and offered to teach him the business. Ken took to it. "Something about it clicked. I never would have thought it would, but it struck a chord. I liked the orderliness." He also liked getting nonjudgmental help and attention from a male relative for the first time in his life.

The third try at college was the charm. Ken did well, went on to law school, and found himself a hot property as a specialist in real estate law ("I had the right stuff for the résumé"). For the first time in his life he had entrée into his father's world. "I went into my career full-force. Behind this was the idea that I could finally make my father happy; it was a link between us. It gave me an identity I could grab onto—'Wow! My father's really proud of me.' I never questioned whether it was what I wanted, and I ended up doing it for twenty years."

Ken was thrilled to speak his father's language at long last—so thrilled that he ignored his own growing sense of self-alienation and depression. The work was compelling and lucrative, and the gratification of meeting his father for lunch and talking business almost compensated for his years of childhood misery. "We had a relationship, and he tried to connect, but I never got past the feeling I'd had since age six that he was bigger than life," Ken said. Like Sherry Taylor's father, Mr. Meredith left no room for his child to create a separate life or to develop convictions of his own. "I was in awe of him; I never believed in myself. Even though I'd reached an impasse and was growing increasingly dissatisfied with the corporate life, the thought never crossed my mind that I could leave it and play music again."

Ken changed his mind once Mr. Meredith suddenly died a month after being diagnosed with a rare heart condition. Although Ken was shocked and devastated ("it was as though God just died"), he found himself playing his drums again a few months later and went to a jam session for the first time in fifteen years. It was immediately clear to him what he was missing. "I was drawn back to what I'd abandoned. I realized I didn't want to go back to the financial world."

At the age of forty-seven, he has returned to his first love, but this time he is pursuing it with all the seriousness and concentration of an independent adult rather than a rebellious adolescent— practicing regularly, building the "right stuff for a résumé" from gigs, and wholeheartedly pursuing a career as a jazz musician. "It still feels selfish," Ken admits, "but I know it's what I need to do. I want to do it right; if it takes three years to figure it out, that's what it will be. I have to see myself through a period of uncertainty, and I'm making progress."

Forsaking business for art, which would have been anathema to his father, was unthinkable during Mr. Meredith's lifetime. "Only after the fact did I realize how strong an influence he was.

If he were still around I never would have considered doing this at my age. I'd still be a little kid upset that my father would be upset. His absence means I don't have to worry about him disapproving, even if he wouldn't have disapproved at all." Freed from the burden of his father's disapproval, even inside his own head, he marches to his own drumbeat at last.

❧

Most people respond to overbearing parents with defiance, compliance, or a combination of the two. But both bad girls and good boys are reacting to agendas set by somebody other than themselves. Maturity comes when you learn to act in your own behalf—whether it involves eventually doing something your parents wanted you to do or becoming a different kind of rebel—one with a real cause. In either case, pleasing them or displeasing them is no longer the point.

When my old college friend Karen Livingston told me that her husband, Randy, had a story for me, I was curious. I'd had dinner with the Livingstons several times in Philadelphia while visiting Karen and found the striking fifty-two-year-old Randy a delightful, if somewhat laconic, companion. With his droll sense of humor, he seemed like a man very much at home in his own skin—relaxed, confident, able to fix anything. I would never have imagined what a trial his earlier life had been, or that his father made Ken Meredith's seem laid-back and supportive.

"Life as I knew it was pretty much mapped out for me," Randy said with characteristic understatement and not a trace of complaint. "My dad was an engineer and he wanted me to be an engineer as well." Wanting a son to follow in your footsteps is not uncommon, nor necessarily pathological, but Mr. Livingston fanatically and relentlessly stage-managed every breath Randy took from elementary school on. "He was always planning what college I'd go to when I wanted to be outside playing baseball." Mr. Livingston was compulsive about his own livelihood as well as his son's future. "We moved a lot, every two years, like army brats, because he kept trying to better himself by changing jobs. We moved from state to state—one of the reasons I'm pretty reserved about reaching out to make friends is because I was always saying good-bye," he said. Randy now understands what drove his father. "He'd worked since the age of ten, and his own father died young so he never knew him well. To keep me from making the same mistakes he'd made himself he forced me a bit and kept on pushing." Mr. Livingston, lacking a positive paternal influence himself, was determined—however misguided his execution—to be a hands-on parent.

Homework in particular became a battle of wills. "He had a regimented, authoritarian way of doing things," Randy recalled. "He used to check what I did every night. We'd go over it, and if I didn't do as good a job as he thought I should, we'd do it over again. I couldn't go out to play with my friends. Eventually you stop fighting and it becomes part of your life. Now I realize he liked it—that little bit of competition." It was also a perverse way to force his son to keep him company. But even then, Randy found ways to hold his own. "I knew he didn't like when I beat him at wrestling; I was physically larger than he was," he said gleefully. Mr. Livingston's plan backfired mightily; all he accomplished was to undermine his highly intelligent son's confidence and make him detest school—and the self-appointed schoolmaster.

When the long-awaited time came for Randy to attend college, it was the last thing he wanted to do. But, like Ken, he chose the route of self-sabotage rather than overt defiance of his father's wishes. "He had it mapped out that I'd go to Purdue and I didn't want to go anywhere, so I just basically gave up and attended the local community college. I've always hated going to school—I hate everything about it—so I made no friends, never spoke to anybody, and got lousy grades." Randy won this round of their mental wrestling match and, over his father's furious objections, dropped out and took a job in a construction company. But because he was still locked into their relationship, he joined the firm of which his father was vice president. There, also like Ken, he found a more sympathetic father figure in the construction superintendent who recognized his talent. "I really had to prove myself as an employee, and it was a double whammy because of my father's position in the company, but I traveled all over the country on jobs with my mentor. I lived in every state, and I proved my mettle. I made it, and got promoted to foreman and superintendent. I showed that I could do it, and that I didn't need the schooling part of it."

Randy's love for Karen, and his decision to marry her even though she had been divorced, finally severed any vestiges of a relationship with his father. When they ran into financial difficulty and had to ask Mr. Livingston to cosign for a loan, Randy felt he had to "crawl." "The wedge between us just got harder and deeper," he said.

Just at the time that his father was exhibiting the first signs of Alzheimer's disease, Randy's fortunes improved dramatically. He got a job working for a competitor of his father's company and rose to the top. Things really started to take off when Randy became an expert in occupational safety, a field he discovered—as his father's painstaking son—that he had a special knack and relish for. "I began doing things I never dreamt I'd be able to do—including wearing a tie to work," he noted—an identification with his father that he could finally tolerate.

Even though Randy was thriving professionally, he recognized that not having a college degree was limiting his opportunities. It was Karen who encouraged him to take the plunge. "She went to college late in life, and when she finished she said, 'OK, it's your turn,'" Randy said. "And I finally did it, as a distance learner. I was able to study; I did all my homework and didn't have anybody check it!" His father had been dead five years.

Randy handled graduation his way. "I chose not to go the ceremony—I didn't even get a ring. I did it on my own terms, and to see the look and the smile on my wife's face. I had a picture taken of myself in my hard hat holding my diploma. I barely made it through high school, and here I was at forty-seven getting my college degree." Sometimes he still can't believe what he has overcome—or that his industry would actually name a workplace safety award for him, as happened recently. Ironically, he has fulfilled his father's dream after all; his official title is "safety engineer."

Randy's self-confidence has developed so profoundly in the years since his father's death that by the time we met it seemed entirely natural. "It was after the fact. I never knew at the time that I was reacting to his death, but I can see that a burden was lifted because of it. I've become more and more positive about myself because it's me making the decisions about my life without worrying what someone else thinks. If I do good, I pat myself on the back, and if I mess up, I have to deal with it." Still, his father's good opinion, even in the hereafter, matters to him; as a child Randy must have perceived some goodwill under that will of iron. "I almost want to say to him, 'Now do you see?'—and I feel like he says 'OK, maybe you did pretty good.' I wish I could show him my name and face on the industry web site, so he could see I've testified for the federal government. At times I think my dad's saying from above, with the wink of an eye and a little grin—'Atta boy.'"

Randy's pride, which he imagines his father finally able to celebrate, came by increments, as any deep change always does. "It didn't happen on the day of his passing—it took a while. I might still have gone back to school if he'd lived, but I would have asked him if it was a good idea and never known on my own. When he was around you never knew that you knew anything. I never thought I could do anything right. It's like waking up and finding out you're as good as Picasso."

⁓

How do some children manage to override the onslaught during the despotic parent's lifetime, while death alone frees others to find their own power? Love has a lot to do with it; less damage is done if there was empathy and concern—however buried—along with the criticism, or if somebody else (the other parent, relatives, teachers, or mentors) provided encouragement. So does temperament; some children are less permeable or more resilient. But the best antidote, whenever in life one attains it, is realizing that your life is your creation and that the only standards worth meeting are your own.

CHAPTER 10

Mom's Best Friend

The End of Emotional Caretaking

When I was in psychoanalytic training, one of my instructors jolted us all by announcing, with a completely straight face, "The best prerequisite for becoming a good therapist is a depressed mother." The whole class laughed in painful recognition because everybody qualified. Each one of us, including me, had been a "child therapist" who had learned the essentials of our eventual profession at home, out of necessity; we had all tried to save our parents, give them solace, ease their pain, figure out and fix what ailed them—daunting tasks that we had accomplished with varying degrees of success. The effort bred patience, sensitivity, and the ability to empathize, but it also caused resentment, anxiety, an overly developed capacity to put our own needs aside or to suppress that we had any in the first place—and underneath the inevitable depression, anger at being picked for the job.

What makes a good psychotherapist also makes a good, if burdened and prematurely mature, daughter; sons can also take care of their mothers, but women more typically turn to their same-sex children to be the mothers they themselves should have had. It also creates a daughter who is ripe to experience profound death benefits when her duties end.

In thirty-five years of psychotherapy practice, I have rarely had a patient who did not spend a significant part of her childhood—and often her adulthood, too—caring for her mother in ways both obvious and subtle. One of them dreamed that she was holding her full-grown mother on her lap like a baby, a physical representation of their psychological relationship. "It seemed odd to be holding a full-grown woman, but I realized that she was perfectly comfortable in that position even though I was not," she wryly observed. Several others literally had to take over and raise their younger siblings in their mother's place. A few were relegated to the tragic role of full-time foster parents, police, or live-in counselors, begging their mothers to stop drinking or shielding them from brutal husbands; one was selected by her family at age eight to take her mother to the mental hospital every time she had a breakdown. But most of them did duty as Mom's Best Friend.

Daughters serve as their mother's confidantes, nurses, witnesses, spouses, publicists, saviors, surrogates, and artistic creations. Some do it literally, like the classmate of mine whose mother picked her up from the school playground at noon every day so they could have lunch together. My own mother never went that far, but she did complain when I was a teenager that I preferred my friends' company to hers—and I felt guilty and disloyal that it was true without recognizing the absurdity of the accusation. In the worst-case scenarios, children are made to feel that their mother's very survival depends on them; this is almost always a blackmail attempt or an act of jealous rage. The mother of a former patient of mine made a suicide attempt while her daughter was on her honeymoon; another patient's mother conveniently had a nervous breakdown every time her daughter, a gifted dancer on the verge of being discovered, had an important audition. Both of these women loved their mothers, but they spent years feeling like unwilling, barely competent saviors. Well into middle age, neither one found it easy to enjoy her life or pursue her talents without keeping one ear open for her mother's cries for help.

Many of the women (and several of the men) I interviewed were emotional caretakers—Carol Costas, who comforted and kept her mother company while her father philandered; Marsha Montgomery, who rushed back to her parents' home in the middle of the night every time her mother had an anxiety attack; and Sharon Black, who protected her mother from feeling like a failure by persevering in a suffocating traditional marriage herself. Beth Grant, the aspiring midlife actress who had spent her youth as the custodian of her mother's fragile self-esteem, had a dream that epitomized the task that burdens many such daughters:

> I was at a restaurant and Martha Stewart was there. Something made me realize that she'd been in prison and I wanted to spare her humiliation, cover her sense of shame. I was making her feel better by going to sit next to her, taking care of her and helping her. Nobody else recognized her; I was the only one who knew who she was.

The toll that sparing your mother and knowing the truth about her takes is often apparent only in retrospect. Beth's mother—who always looked put together on the surface like Martha Stewart but who was imprisoned in desperate unhappiness all her life—was dead two years before her daughter could have this insightful dream about her own role in her mother's life. It is hard indeed to have had such an assignment and not feel guilty at the immensity of your relief when you can finally eat out in peace.

Parental caretaking is not all bad and certainly not all pathological; it is built into being human; research shows that babies are already consoling adults with reassuring pats by the age of one. But when sustaining your mother takes precedence over living your life, or when doing so is compulsive, oppressive, or depressing, it becomes role reversal, not loving empathy. A parent who is unable to acknowledge or reciprocate a child's efforts oppresses her child. This can happen even when they love each other dearly; all relationships have a dark side.

❧

My colleague Laura Reynolds certainly met the painful professional qualification my teacher had specified; her father had died the day she was born, and her devastated mother remained depressed through most of Laura's childhood. Although we'd known each other for years, Laura lived in Long Island and I rarely saw her; she never attended or presented papers at professional meetings and gave the impression that her clinical practice was not the focus of her attention. It was always a pleasure when we did meet, though; beneath her self-effacing manner she was funny, warm, and sharp.

"I never would have thought there was anything good about her death until the topic of your book came up," she told me when we spoke. "For me, it was 95 percent loss and only five percent benefit." But she also recognized that the positive consequences of her becoming an orphan, though subtle and internal, were profound and life-changing.

"My mother and I had a very close and not very conflicted relationship," she said. "When you grow up with only one parent and the other dies young, you're much more connected to the one you have left." There was, however, one potential source of conflict that Laura arranged her life in order to circumvent: "My mother had been offered a scholarship to Johns Hopkins University and her father refused to allow her to accept it, so she was always concerned about her lack of a college education. When I got my PhD I was very proud and happy—and she made one very telling comment: 'You didn't have to go *that* far.' It was too much for her; all that competitive stuff was there underneath. In her mind it was just too large a gulf between us, though I didn't think so at the time."

Even though Laura claims not to have considered the achievement gulf between them as yawning as her mother did, she took unconscious pains to narrow it by making her life as much like her mother's as possible. "Over time I became aware that I'd been placing emphasis elsewhere, like in family life. I never gave my career 100 percent—not that I didn't pursue it, but I didn't have the success I could have had." While her mother was alive, she held herself back without realizing it, explaining her self-imposed professional limitations as a lack of ability rather than an avoidance of conflict. "I didn't see myself putting the kind of time into my work that other people I knew did, so I thought maybe I wasn't as good as they were. I was completely comfortable about this." Laura was comfortable because curbing her ambition preempted any possible discord and protected their bond. Supporting her mother's self-esteem and preventing strife took precedence over her own professional fulfillment.

Things changed—seemingly without conscious effort—after Laura's mother died ten years ago, when Laura was fifty-one.

Laura's mother had been a subliminal impediment to her daughter's ambition since the day she uttered her fateful comment; after her death, when the comparison between their achievements was no longer relevant or hurtful, Laura implicitly gave herself permission to excel. "The professional side of my life suddenly became extra easy for me. I was too late for certain things, but I branched out in other directions. I became very active in the hierarchical structure of my church, and I had a full-time practice simultaneously. I have felt free to do whatever I wanted in a way that was quite mysterious to me until you told me what you were writing about. I realized that what made the difference in my life was that I don't have to worry about her feelings anymore. As a result I participate in my professional life much more comfortably—not necessarily doing different things, but feeling differently about it." Now that she is free from the fear that she could hurt or anger her mother, she has no need to hold herself back. As a result, she appreciates her own talent and makes full use of it. "Today I definitely feel that I'm very good. I know that if I wanted to go out and get active in the field, to run for office or be in the public eye, I could do it with confidence." Since she no longer has to worry about the gulf, she can rise to any heights she wants.

Any daughter whose mother is widowed young feels special sympathy and connection with her, but some connections are more dangerous—literally as well as figuratively—than others. Like Laura Reynolds, Jennifer Sloan also lost her father in early childhood and had to deal with her mother's despair afterward. But Jennifer's mother never got over it and remained "completely dependent" on her for the rest of her life. Jennifer was even closer to her mother than Laura was to hers—far too close. Even though Mrs. Sloan became a political organizer for the women's liberation movement, her daughter was her ballast. "She had no friends but me," Jennifer said, "and she never went out with a man again. I was her best friend forever and she was mine." The mother turned out to be a more problematic friend than the daughter did.

Jennifer, a forty-seven-year-old graphic designer, had volunteered to participate in my research, but the first thing she said when I called to arrange an interview was, "I don't know if I fit"; to declare on the record that her mother's death three years previously had done her any good made her uneasy. In order to protect her mother's reputation (and her own positive feelings), she acted as her posthumous press agent, sending me in advance an extensive biography that listed her mother's accomplishments in glowing terms and enumerated the famous people she had known. Her feelings about her mother were more contradictory, and more threatening, than she had any idea.

Although Jennifer insisted that Mrs. Sloan was "utterly devoted" to her—"I never had a minute's doubt that I was second only to the Messiah in her eyes," she declared—she also told me a dreadful story about her childhood. "My mother confessed to me that after my father's death she had wanted to bundle me into the car and drive into a wall, but she hadn't done it because she was afraid I might live. It was an act of love," she concluded, whitewashing the shocking aggression inherent in both her mother's intention and her announcement. "She wanted to spare me the pain of living after my father was dead." That it might be at least as painful for Jennifer if only her mother had died in the attempt to kill them both did not occur to Mrs. Sloan since they could not be parted: their identities were fused in her mind. Decades later Jennifer was still denying her mother's chilling insensitivity and lack of boundaries, excusing them as excessive maternal solicitude.

She felt compelled to justify her mother's decision not to commit murder and suicide—and also to prevent a lethal change of heart—by dedicating her life to her best friend's well-being.

Mrs. Sloan was an avid champion for the rights of every woman except her own daughter, and Jennifer, out of love and fear, never questioned her expectations. She invited her mother along on every vacation she and her husband took—even when they were trying to conceive a child. "I thought that being a good daughter meant including her in everything," she explained. Filial "duty" trumped every other right and responsibility.

Though she still feels guilty admitting it, Jennifer knows that surviving her mother has done her good. "My mother was all about herself. She could not separate my emotions from hers; having a child was a big mistake for her. I don't have to get sucked into her intensity or demands any longer," she admitted. Still, she is compelled to add, "Nobody gives me pep talks like she did."

The impermeable boundary that death has imposed between them is Jennifer's biggest benefit. Being the one left alive—the fate her mother wanted to "spare" her—enables her to separate her own emotions from her mother's; she could create a one-person rather than a two-person identity. But to do so, she must come to terms with a mother whose personality was a potent mixture of impressive and destructive, inspiring and engulfing. "Her death has made me understand all the work I have ahead of me, all of the time I've lost," she said. Acknowledging and grieving for her losses begin that work.

❧

Sons also become their mothers' compulsive caretakers. They face the same guilt, resentment, obligation, and anxiety that daughters do, with the additional shame of feeling like unmasculine, dependent "Momma's Boys." The demise of such a mother lets her son become a man.

Forty-six-year-old Kevin Peterson had an older brother and sister, but he was chosen, and accepted the assignment, as his mother's full-time, live-in attendant for the last seven years of her life. He quit his job in the cable television industry and moved back to the house where he was born to care for her after she was diagnosed with cancer. On the first anniversary of her death, Kevin contacted me with an unusual worry: "I'm concerned," he said, "that I'm taking her death TOO well."

"We were very close and had a very good relationship, but I was her primary caretaker and I realize in hindsight how stressful it was," he explained. "I did anything and everything for her, so I have the blessing of peace of mind and not a scintilla of regret. I was beside myself right after she died, but what's troubling me now is how liberated I feel—have I dissociated from her? Is this a post-traumatic reaction? Should I be in therapy? If I'm really at peace about it, am I just creating a problem?" Kevin's problem was real, but it was different than he thought; he was actually struggling with the same sense of lost time and buried rage that plagued Jennifer Sloan.

When I asked what made him feel so uncomfortably liberated, Kevin responded, "My life is more my own to do with as I please. I have more right to it since I don't have to report to her. That wasn't true when I lived with her, and I told her so. I was always concerned that if I went out for the evening, she'd have a fall; she'd make a face if she heard that I'd made plans to go out." He complained, but he stayed home.

The degree to which Kevin allowed his mother's displeasure to control him suggested that he was an unofficial mother's helper long before he became an official one. "I was always more attuned to her than my siblings were," he said. "I never was good at setting boundaries. My mother was unhappy with her husband and looked to me. I could never stand to see her hurt; as a child nothing tore me asunder more than seeing her cry, and as an adult there was still that little boy in me that couldn't tolerate it." Severely limiting his own emotional and physical mobility was the price he paid to prevent her tears. For some sensitive children, their mother's distress is like a telephone ringing; it has a "demand quality" that they may resent but cannot ignore.

Kevin feels victimized by his mother, but he realizes that he colluded with her, and that the arrangement served both their needs. "She enabled me because it was to her benefit to keep me down. Fear held me back, and I grew complacent. Taking care of her became a safe haven from the rest of the world, a way to find purpose and meaning in my life; I was willing to put up with all the negative stuff rather than say it wasn't healthy," he admitted.

Now that he no longer has any place to hide, he sees both the opportunities and the obstacles that lay before him. "Finally I can go out at midnight for a three-hour walk and not be greeted at the door and told that it's dangerous," he said. "I don't miss being infantilized, but I'll never have back those seven years. Being there was a vicious cycle—the longer I was out of work, the less employable I became. How am I going to explain it on a résumé? I'm scared to death about my future."

Kevin has taken a major step to becoming an adult by accepting responsibility for putting his life entirely at his mother's disposal. "Hiding in her house and as her caretaker for all those years makes me angry at myself; I put it at my own doorstep. Even though I don't know how to grow up, it's a position I embrace. Twenty years ago I would have thought that the day she died would have been the worst of my life, but it was just the opposite."

~⁀⌒⁀~

However much you may have hated the job of keeping your mother afloat, losing that job is disorienting; a lifetime of focusing on someone else's needs makes it hard to determine or pursue your own when you finally get the opportunity in middle age. The death of an emotionally dependent parent is always a relief to the caretaker-child—often guilty relief—but it is also troubling that you felt you had to do it for so long and at such great personal cost. And, inevitably, it is sad.

Beth Grant, like Jennifer Sloan and Kevin Peterson, could never say no to her mother. After too many years serving as an audience, becoming an actress feels like a necessity to Beth—so much so that she intends to take an early retirement from the Boston Board of Education to pursue her new vocation as soon as possible. Recognizing that she could never have dared to consider such a step until her mother died filled her with a poignant combination of sorrow, fear, and exhilaration.

"Ownership of my life feels so luxurious, but it's also terrifying because this is the first time I've done anything for myself. While my mother was alive I could never even imagine retiring. Acting wasn't a possibility because I couldn't stop teaching—it was the only independence I had. That's one of the things I have to grieve for.

"After my father died, my mother used to say, 'Quit your job and move back in with me.' As long as I was still working I could always say, 'I can't come over because I have a class to teach'—I could use that obligation to avoid rejecting her." Beth had so thoroughly internalized her mother's point of view that she actually believed she was a bad, abandoning daughter if she wanted to do anything (including doing nothing at all) outside her mother's aegis. Because she did not believe she had a right to self-determination, working was the only acceptable excuse, the only way to prevent herself from completely capitulating to her mother's demands. She and Kevin Peterson both avoided addressing their own problems by keeping their mothers at the center of the universe. "I always knew what I had to do," Beth said. "I didn't have to deal with loneliness, or disappointment, or structure time for myself because she came first. It was comforting not to have to make changes in my life, and it was safe." It was safe, but it was not living.

Her mother's death made Beth's ploy to get herself off the hook both impossible and unnecessary; when the telephone stops ringing, you don't have to find excuses not to answer it. "I can't use anything external as a reason for not meeting other people's needs anymore because nobody needs me," she said. "I'm no longer controlled by outside forces—success or failure is all mine from now on. It's freeing and also scary to grab onto my life." Beth's retirement as her mother's handmaiden is her debut as the mistress of her destiny.

When a daughter comes to terms with having spent her life as her mother's best friend, she becomes the best friend she really needs: her own.

PART IV

In Morte Veritas

The Insights Death Brings

CHAPTER 11

THE ELEVENTH HOUR

Near-Death Revelations

༄

"I love teaching people who have lost their parents how to write sonnets," my poet friend says. "I call the last line, the fourteenth, the 'deadline,' because you've got to work it all out by then; it's your last chance to resolve everything that came before." The sense of urgency she communicates to her students is not desperation but a call to marshal the concentrated effort and attention that creative conclusions require.

Nature imitates art. When a parent's death is imminent, either because of a diagnosis or age or your inability to deny the reality of mortality any longer, you reach the deadline of the relationship. Deadlines should be taken very seriously. The eleventh hour—the last years, or months, or even minutes of a parent's life—is your final opportunity for direct communication. This transitional period between adulthood with living parents and orphanhood is also the time to cultivate readiness for the insights and changes that losing a mother or father will make possible.

Unless a parent dies without warning, most of us are conscious when we enter the peri-death space. I knew that my father was dying when I was thirty-two, but my state of mind made me miss the opportunity entirely. I tried to detach myself from the process because of the strains in our relationship, so we were both deprived of meaningful contact until I remedied that retroactively by writing about us twenty years later. My anguished regret made me particularly determined not to repeat the mistake.

My mother survived him by twenty-five years, and by then I was a different person. I remember the exact moment I entered that zone with her. When I learned that she had early Alzheimer's disease, I felt the weight of the world literally descend onto my shoulders; in addition to the crushing caretaking responsibilities I suddenly faced, I felt instantly compelled to communicate with her in some meaningful way while there was still time. During the endgame I also vowed to make as much sense of our relationship as possible, whether she participated or not—as she did, miraculously, from her deathbed.

Patients often come to me with a similar agenda: to work through their relationship with an aging parent, usually a mother, while they still can. "I don't want her to die while I'm still so furious at her," they plead—and usually they succeed; the prospect of a funeral concentrates the mind. Although reconciliation and acknowledgment are what most people long for, there are other routes to resolution with parents. Even if a parent cannot or will not engage, a child can. When Alice Gerard approached her mother in the hospital, she refused to discuss their relationship and the incest she had failed to prevent; yet Alice (who later wrote about helping her beloved dog die) was able to grieve for her and forgive her because, as she said, "I did it by myself in therapy."

Some breakthroughs occur at the eleventh hour, and only then—words spoken or exchanged that reverberate forever and shared experiences beyond words. Some of the most important transformations come from troubling insights about conflicted relationships considered in solitude. The resolutions children create, with or without their parents' assistance, were unimaginable before.

Tammy Carter, a sixty-three-year-old physical therapist and yoga instructor, detested her mother her whole life, and the feeling was mutual. "From childhood on, our relationship was venomous and vitriolic. She hated me and neglected me," the vivacious redhead told me. Mrs. Carter had children only at the insistence of her husband and considered Tammy, whom he adored, her rival from the day she was born; she didn't treat her son, Tammy's younger brother, well, either, but she did not reject him as cruelly. She blamed Tammy for Mr. Carter's sudden death at age forty-two; in her opinion, he had killed himself by working so hard to lavish the little girl with presents. "After he died there was a bitter war between us, and we didn't speak for years," Tammy said. She left home at seventeen, "unforgiving and intending to remain so."

When Tammy became a middle-aged woman herself, she made efforts to empathize with her mother and attempted to reconcile with her but was rebuffed every time. Tammy didn't even get a card for her fiftieth birthday, which she took as confirmation that her mother regretted having given birth to her in the first place. But Tammy knew that hating her mother took a toll on her, and she vowed to neutralize it if she could. "My relationship with her was the worst wound I had, and changing it was my project," she said.

Five years later, Tammy's mother had the first in a series of increasingly debilitating strokes, and once again Tammy tried to reach her, this time in her professional capacity. The role reversal worked like a charm. "I acted as a physical therapist, not a child; I put on my little white uniform in my head and took care of her. When she recovered, she came back as someone else—she still had her hateful temper and vicious tongue, but there was another, better person inside." The daughter intuitively chose a nonverbal route to this new person. "I got her to go in the swimming pool and push me in an inner tube. We laughed and played like we had never done in my entire life, like we were friends." Her face lit up as she savored the memory; in her mother's second childhood, Tammy had retrieved something she had never gotten before.

Each stroke brought the mother and daughter closer, and Tammy's compassion grew as her mother's ability to hurt her waned. "She became less and less able and more and more appreciative, more dependent on my assistance. There were even fleeting moments when I thought I loved this person. I also saw how my brother was totally disabled by his rage. He was becoming angrier and more bitter all the time, and only wanted her to die—all he could do was write checks." Her brother's response provided an instructive counterexample that motivated her even more. A sibling's reactions, however destructive or immature, can give you perspective.

In the last three years of her mother's life, it became Tammy's mission to sustain her, and she shuttled regularly from her home in Vermont to the nursing home in Texas where her mother, who had managed to alienate practically everybody in her life, languished. "She'd look like hell, like she was dead, when I arrived," Tammy recalled. "So I'd sing to her, wash her hair and paint her nails. I made her come back to life, and she was so grateful." By reviving her mother, Tammy turned the tables in a remarkable way, giving back the very thing her mother had begrudged her.

The words she had always longed to hear, and to speak, were her reward. "I'll never forget our last visit. She hadn't talked for three weeks and was being tube fed. I got her up, put on her makeup, made her eat and laugh; I forced her to relate, and I enjoyed her company. By the end of the day she actually smiled at me! 'I'll be back in a few days,' I said. Then I said 'I love you'— and for the first time in my life I meant it. She looked at me and she said to me, 'I'll miss you every day.' I threw my arms around her, and we both cried. It was the last time I saw her." In the midst of death, she created love.

Taking care of a parent at the end of life, a task that fills most people with dread, can have surprising consequences. The longed-for tearful embrace that Tammy and her mother had the good fortune to share is one possibility; confronting a troubling truth you never recognized before is another, equally enriching outcome.

Sam Whitman and I were friends as teenagers. He seemed to lead a charmed life; he was deep; articulate; socially adept; and, so I imagined, untouched by angst. He lived in a rambling house in a gracious neighborhood (his mother was from a wealthy family), and his father was a renowned liberal Christian theologian with a reputation as an exceptional teacher and a coterie of acolytes. When we met again after our fortieth high school reunion, I discovered that I had correctly remembered his sensitivity and intelligence—we could have talked all day—but that the serenity and self-possession I had attributed to him were my own projections. I also learned that he had experienced what he described as "a true epiphany, a sudden key to my life that allowed me to become more myself" through caring for his dying parents.

My family traumas were more dramatic than Sam's, but his had hidden effects at least as serious. The difference was that, while I had known the truth for years, he didn't have a clue that anything was amiss until he was in his midfifties; before that, he had bought the family myth that all was well and had assumed that he himself was the problem ("I was stupid and lazy"). Becoming his parents' physical caretaker suddenly made him realize that he had been performing that function psychologically his entire life.

Managing his parents' lives was déjà vu all over again for Sam. "When I became the general contractor for their upkeep as their health began to fail—I buried my ambivalence and encouraged them to come live near me—I watched them become literally the children they had always been emotionally. I saw that I had been responsible for their care and feeding throughout my childhood, and how much I'd resented it. It was a terrible, intrusive burden, and very hard work." The hardest part of Sam's lifelong job had been bolstering his father's ego by sabotaging and denigrating his own talents—especially the ones father and son shared.

"Although I've had many moments of missing my parents, I was relieved when they died," Sam said with refreshing frankness. "It still feels disloyal to say these things—what if they're someplace where they can hear me? I've revised a lot of what I thought, and come to appreciate startling negatives in my upbringing. As a result I have a more complete view of my parents, especially of my father. Curiously, I can recall my love with less distress now that I have discovered what a prison I was raised in when he was the warden."

The image of this beloved religious leader as his son's jailer was hard to fathom—I had heard him speak once and still remember his sparkling eyes and charismatic presence—but Sam now laid out the painful truth of his childhood for me, the truth he had only started putting together five years ago in the penumbra of his parents' deaths; not to connect the dots when you can't stand to know what shape they will reveal is a common defensive maneuver. "My mother made me her emotional companion; she confessed to me that she had stopped loving him three months after they were married. I did love my father—I remember hugging him and the way he smelled—but I never liked or respected him, both because of his actions and his values."

It was Dr. Whitman's arrogance and, especially, his veniality, so discordant with his persona and his religious principles, that repelled his son. "My father was obsessed with money. He portrayed himself as a math wiz and an expert in economics. He used to brag about his success as an investor, and he spent hours every day poring over the stock pages"—an avocation financed entirely by his wife's inheritance. "He was infantile, always complaining about missed opportunities and blaming his brokers for giving him poor advice and thwarting his ability to make millions more in the market. To the end of his life he regretted that he wasn't wealthier."

As a result, Sam ran in the other direction; somehow, he managed to graduate from Yale and the University of Chicago Law School without thinking he was smart. "Because I had to advertise to myself and to the world that my father was the brilliant scholar, I thought I wasn't any good at school—especially at math. It was easy for me, but I often made 'careless' errors that sabotaged my grades. As a result my academic career was highly erratic. Now I realize I was conflicted; I actually love math. I avoided studying economics, and I couldn't read the financial pages—they always swam before my eyes. My father made fun of this and gently characterized me as someone who would never make money."

Sam's father's gentle chiding masked competitiveness so insidious that it was undetectable, and that did not stop until he was incapacitated. "I was only able to discuss finances with him—knowledgebly—right before he died," Sam told me. "That was when I figured out that I'd denied a good bit of who I was just to avoid being like him. Now it's clear to me that I was in fact a competent entrepreneur and businessman—I started a law firm specializing in civil rights, one of the largest of its kind in the U.S., and for twenty-five years I managed it, including creating budgets for a sizable staff, thinking all the time that I was hopeless in money matters. I never added up that I was actually a financial success." To calculate accurately his own achievements would have raised questions about his father's assessment of him that he had been unwilling to address.

Sam wanted so much to escape from the paternal sphere of influence that he also denied his own scholarly bent. "I couldn't wait to leave school and plunge into the arena of action and social change," he said. The profession he chose reflected his father's liberal politics while avoiding the taint of his father's greed.

But supervising his father's last years made it possible for Sam to repossess in middle age aspects of himself that he had repudiated. He turned the firm he had created over to younger colleagues; moved cross-country; and just like his father, became a teacher and a scholar in his own field. "While he was alive, the thought of any permanent position in academia seemed repugnant to me. After his death I did what I never could have imagined: I became a professor and an academic, teaching legal economics, and I love it."

Sam knows that insight doesn't fix everything. "There is no doubt that my father's death and dying permitted me to embrace aspects of myself that resembled him and that I had previously denied. I still have trouble with the stock pages, though; they still swim. My investments do fine anyway." But he doesn't pout, or tout himself as a badly advised genius, if they don't.

Facing the truth about his father allowed Sam to integrate his father's best qualities into his own life; he discovered the curative power of seeing a parent whole. "Confronting these issues unraveled the knot of unconsciousness inside me, so that I could express my negative feelings. Only then could I access the love I still felt for him—the primitive, physical love, different from admiration or forgiveness—with less conflict. His dying revitalized my life."

❧

Sam came into his own by finally facing his father's worst qualities. Peter Sawyer's tender care of a father who had showed him little but his worst qualities until the end allowed him to discover his own masculine power at last.

Peter, the man who seemed to have been dropped into his working-class family from another planet, has been my massage therapist for twenty years. I've enjoyed his wit; admired his aesthetic sense; and relied on his empathic, powerful, curative touch through many crises. One night, he told me how he had used his healing hands to console his father during his final hours.

"My father was a raging alcoholic for most of my adult life," he said in his quiet, straightforward way. "He never hugged me growing up; he had vowed not to touch his children because his own father had been physically violent." Peter's father, a factory worker, was intimidated by his son's intellect and belittled him for his utter lack of mechanical ability, but they shared a love of nature. "We did have our moments when I was a child; it was touching. He let me be creative and attended my concerts when I sang in the chorus. Although he built me a tree house in his basement workshop, he used to teach woodworking to the neighborhood kids, never to me." Peter was hungry for a connection that he did not have the requisite skills to make.

Mr. Sawyer began drinking heavily in Peter's adolescence and started to humiliate him when he figured out that his son was gay. With rage, shame, and sorrow, Peter remembers having to carry him into the house when he came home drunk, a regular occurrence. One night, after pouring all the liquor in the house down the drain, the twenty-five-year-old left home for good and vowed never to speak to his father again as long as he kept drinking. "We never made up and never discussed it," Peter said, and he assumed that they would always be estranged. Relieved of the burden of trying to please his father, Peter left his desk job at the phone company—the job his father approved of—and became a massage therapist, a profession that would have excited nothing but contempt from his macho parent. Then, when Peter was in his forties, his father finally quit drinking; "he realized that he was unconscious and wanted to be conscious."

Even though the tension between the changeling son and the uncomprehending father never completely dissipated, they began to spend time together in silent communion. "He liked to just sit with me when I came to visit. We'd go outside, build a fire, and he'd get me coffee without saying a word. We'd watch storms come in together, and he'd teach me about birds, just like we used to do when I was a little kid." Nature was the language they had in common.

Then Peter's father got leukemia. He had been ill for months and refused to see a doctor until Peter insisted on taking him. Half a year later he was on his deathbed, with his son sitting silently beside him. "Although he never complained, I realized he was in terrible pain; for the first time in my life I saw him crying." To take care of the man he now loved, Peter employed the skill his father had never approved of. "He was so tortured. I wanted to comfort him, so I gave him a leg and foot massage. I'd never touched him before." Then, the son broke the silence between them. "I told him he was dying, that it was OK. I told him I'd take care of my mother, to just go. I gave him permission to die. I tried to soothe him, and I think I was able to relieve him."

Touching his father at the very end—they were both good with their hands, as it turned out—showed him a fact that had been hidden for years. "He and I were a lot closer than we ever talked about. One thing came to light after our reconciliation: I actually liked my father more than my mother. I really came to appreciate him and to take on his masculinity. I feel stronger now, much more myself." Therapeutic touch, which his father had been too afraid to bestow himself, established Peter as a loving, effective man in his own right.

The deadline may not be the last chance to resolve everything, but it is the beginning of a new chapter if you make it so.

CHAPTER 12

PERSPECTIVES FROM THE DEATHSPACE

᮪ꢚꣲ

Brave New World

The Deathspace, where survivors reconsider the dead, is a unique vantage point, a state of mind so real it seems like a physical location. Orphans go there most and know it best.

Things look different from the Deathspace. Before you arrive, you cannot imagine the features of the landscape that will unfold before your mind's eye. People, including yourself, suddenly come into focus as never before. You see more deeply and more clearly, and you know that what you see is true; this new perspective changes you forever. From a curative distance, parents become fellow human beings, less powerful and more poignant, and you become their peer. The Deathspace is the final frontier of the parent/child relationship, where authentic adulthood emerges and death benefits are born.

This evocative place-name was coined by Jan Kahn, the gay woman whose mother had shunned her and only partially reconciled with her during her agonizing last illness. Jan told me how, five years later, she discovered in her mother's jewelry box the note of apology the dying woman had written for her to find. She described what happened:

> The "Deathspace" gave me the separation I needed to look at my mother as a person, as somebody who'd become what she was the same way I became who I was—because of her parents and her history. Years earlier, when my mother's sister was in the hospital dying of cancer, my grandmother—a more controlling woman even than my mother—had told my mother not to visit her (she had a phobia about catching the disease). My mother, who was living at home at the time, listened to her, and never forgave herself. This haunted her right before she died in her own excruciating pain; this was the anguish that she couldn't tell me about, the unbearable guilt that her sister had died totally alone, and in just as much pain. She was so devastated by her conviction that her own suffering was retribution for abandoning her sister that she could focus on nothing else. This was where my mother came from; this was her story. That space after her death enabled me to stop thinking that her rejection was just about me-me-me. I was able to look at her in a more nuanced way. I can live with it now.

Realizations like Jan's are not uncommon; a striking number of bereaved adults use spatial and temporal metaphors to explain the shift in their psychic position vis-à-vis their parents and their past. Deathspaces are also intensely personal, and the people who enter them describe their experience with their own special language.

Joe Bailey, the historian whose dream about his mother's loving arms brought him back to his Catholic faith, saw both his parents through a humane prism after their deaths, the edges of their character flaws smoothed by time. "Now they're in the position of people whose biographies you read," he said. "By dying they free you to appreciate them so completely, with a kind of empathy that would have been impossible to sustain in their lifetimes. I was able to restore them to their full humanity, and to reconstruct their imaginations in a way that couldn't be entertained earlier." He even permitted himself to wonder, with total suspension of judgment, whether his adored mother ever had love affairs.

Ellen Wagner, the artist who became anorectic because her father criticized her weight and everything else about her, said, "I see the dynamics of our relationship from a totally different vantage point since his death; a softness has come into my paintings." I am familiar with Ellen's canvases, and have noticed how tenderness has replaced some of the torment and suppressed violence her earlier work exuded.

A patient of mine with an abstract turn of mind used an algebraic simile to depict the shift in his view of his mother, whom he considered powerful and authoritative during her lifetime and later came to see as childish and hysterical. "Her death was like resolving a fraction. When you take a complicated equation and cancel out all the fractions from it, you don't have a big jumble of numbers and variables anymore—you can just clean it up."

Beth Grant, the English teacher and actress, used a literary metaphor. "You can't make sense of a story—their story—until it ends. Of course it goes on, but then it goes on in you." The dramatis personae stay put at the end of real life as well as in fiction, and this fact makes closure and insight possible. After the finale, children can appreciate the trajectory of their parents' lives and recognize their own roles as characters in the family drama.

In my own case the effect of entering the Deathspace was revolutionary. Even after spending much of my adult life trying to unravel my relationship with my mother, and exerting particular effort during what I knew were the last years of her life, there was a qualitative change in the clarity of my "vision" starting on the day she died. The metaphor I employed was literal; I inserted my own lenses in her glass frames, in an effort to see in a new, integrated way. The lens(es) through which I perceived became wider-angled and my perspective—the derivation of the word is "seeing through and into"—expanded as distance opened up between us, as though a light went on in the dark. This experience has been repeated in the years since she died, each revelation adding to the last, surprising and enlightening me.

What felt like an automatic, almost involuntary experience of being catapulted into a unique state of consciousness was at least partially the product of planning. The receptive state of mind I tried to cultivate assisted me; a similar process allows patients in therapy to have and to recall significant dreams when they're ready to grasp their meaning. Revelations come to some fortunate surviving children without much obvious effort on their parts— but why leave something so important to luck? My insights— both the sudden and the incremental ones—were hard-won, built on a foundation I had carefully laid down while my mother was alive, one which I keep reinforcing. I also hoped and expected to see things differently after her death. Whenever you reach the

Deathspace, you should acknowledge that you have arrived somewhere remarkable. Otherwise it's possible to miss the view.

Detachment and separation, which psychologists used to consider the primary criteria for mental health after mourning, are the hallmarks of how people think in the Deathspace. This type of disengagement is not cold but full of feeling. You do not detach from the story that, as Beth Grant says, "then goes on inside you," but from being entrenched in your own interpretation of that story. Understanding the world from a viewpoint other than your own, the objective state of mind that Jan describes as "not just me-me-me," is a mature accomplishment. Often it enables a child to empathize with—or at least to comprehend—a problematic parent for the first time.

❧

Argentina-born Anita Suarez's Deathspace was literal and physical, and it took her years to get there. The sixty-seven-year-old social worker felt so controlled by her mother's pervasive and malignant power ("I was her dancing puppet, like a doll on a music box moving to a tune that somebody else decides," she said) that she had to put the entire Western Hemisphere between them; she moved from Buenos Aires to Seattle in her twenties and never looked back. Anita did, however, need to look inside her mother's closed casket at her funeral to "make sure she was in there—it was a relief for me."

Anita's mother had rejected her virtually since her birth—an aversion, Anita speculated, that had its origins in her resemblance to her mother's despised first husband. "We were always at odds," she recalled. "I didn't look right in her eyes. I was a dark-eyed brunette, like my father, and she kept trying to lighten my hair. I felt invisible to her. I used to be silent, shy and withdrawn, and she told me I was clumsy. At the time of her death I was attempting to repair our relationship but she wouldn't let me near her; she actually wrote me out of the will. She always had a thing about me."

To feel lovable, attractive, and valuable when your mother hates you is no easy matter, and Anita struggled to feel she deserved a good life; "I always felt guilty about being who I was," she said. Eventually, the silent, awkward child found a welcoming home in her adopted country and grew into an expressive, graceful adult. Years of therapy helped her claim her voice as a singer, her body as a tango dancer, and her sense of value as a provider of public health services for women. But she felt a need to reengage safely with the unmaternal mother who had so possessed her; she knew she had to find a way to resurrect their relationship. "It's not as simple as 'Hooray, the witch is dead!'" Anita said wisely. "The issue is, how do you move on? I resisted her enormously, but when you resist that's all you get. I don't do that now; it's actually kind of remarkable."

Insight and a changed perspective sometimes happen soon after a parent dies but can also take decades to achieve. Leaving her "motherland" during her mother's lifetime and creating a life of her own far away was Anita's first tentative step toward utilizing her Deathspace. Paradoxically, the phobic act of checking that her mother was truly dead at her funeral was the second step; it reassured her of a separation that never felt real before. But if her efforts had stopped there, she would still be in a state of repudiating, rather than integrating, her childhood experience, and she would stay alienated from parts of herself as a result; a parent who is shunned still has power over you.

Anita was ready to go further only when she had reached an age older than her mother had been when she died; outliving her mother reinforced their separateness. It was also a healthy victory that made her feel powerful in her own right. Then, just four years ago, on her mother's birthday, she took the third, definitive step. Now a confident woman rather than a puppet, she could meet her adversary face-to-face at last and call the tune herself:

> I did a ritual with candles and wrote her a letter. I told her what she would like to know, what could impress her and be important to her. "I'm in Seattle," I told her. "I've learned to sing. I dance too, and I'm good at it, and when I get dressed up and go out I feel like a million dollars." And I also said, "Some of my ability to do this came from you." Now I look in the mirror, I see my feet and ankles, and see a little bit of her. I never could do that while she was alive, but now if she could see me, she would think, "Ah yes, this is my girl." It's a gigantic change for me to be willing to do this.

Anita understands that this remarkable transformation—her ability to embody the best of someone who had been so toxic—was possible because her mother was dead; her physical absence from the world was a prerequisite for a safe rapprochement. "The most important thing about death is that part of the loss means locating the person somewhere else and knowing they're not going to come back," she said. "Every day I can have either the sense that she's always with me or that she's not. I can say other women are not my mother, and I am aware that other women can be just like her. Recently I was able to leave a woman therapist who I realized was hostile to me. My mother's relocated; she's not everywhere now. She's in that box, underground, controllable, less pervasive. She's over there and she can't meddle. I can think for myself. I can explore. And, in retrospect, I can even explore her." Her experience in the Deathspace, extreme as it was, is true for all of us.

❧

Some people come to the Deathspace on their own under even the most difficult circumstances; others need help getting there. Usually therapists, friends, or family members provide it. The Johnson sisters got life-changing assistance from two strangers: the funeral director and the priest who acted as confessor to their vicious father.

Neither Sandy nor Linda Johnson had seen their father for twenty-five years, and both of them were relieved that he was out of their lives for good, when their aunt told them he was dying. Sandy, the nomadic executive who later bought a house of her own, was forty-five at the time. She insisted that her younger sister, Linda, whom she had virtually raised, come with her to confront him. Linda had told her several years earlier that their father had raped her when she was four years old—"he used me as a garbage can" was the way she described it—and Sandy felt it was essential that they both be at his deathbed. "I was driven to go and to bring her with me," she said.

As they approached the end of their seventeen-hour journey to the Florida hospital where he lay, Sandy "had a ball of worms in [my] stomach," and Linda, then thirty-eight years old, collapsed in terror. "I was so frightened that I had trouble breathing," she remembered. "He was such a monster in our lives." What they found there was appalling in a different way than they expected. "He was already unconscious when we arrived, and he looked worse than my grandfather," Sandy said.

"It was such a shock; he was horribly old and feeble, and I was still seeing him as all-powerful, as he was in his thirties," Linda added. "I felt a wave of hatred come over me, deep, horrible, and black; it was scary to recognize I had that capacity. I started praying not to carry that ugliness inside anymore. He was dying penniless and alone; there was nothing worse that I could do to him that he hadn't already done to himself. I saw him die. It was a benefit to see that terrifying fiend no longer alive, and I left feeling much safer—I'd been so afraid of him that I'd never even wanted him to know my married name or address. I no longer feel hatred because I know he's really gone; I wouldn't have been freed from that if I hadn't been there to watch it."

Sandy, too, described witnessing his death as "a turning point" that removed her fear and left her "lighthearted." Seeing the dead body of the enemy who should have been their protector provided revenge and comfort for them both, as it did for Anita Suarez. And like her, they were able to go even further.

Despite their relief, the sisters felt deprived of the closure they had come for. "I wondered, 'why are we here?'" Linda said. They went to the funeral home, paid for his funeral, and were preparing to leave town when the funeral director told them that the priest who had confessed their father and spent the last week with him wanted urgently to speak to them. Linda described the three-way conversation. "I said no twice, but he handed me the phone. We talked for an hour; I will never forget what the priest said: 'Your father very deeply regretted the damage he did to you, because he loved you so much. He was haunted by chemical and emotional demons all his life—he had been a drunk since the age of sixteen—and he wasn't able to overcome them.' I lost it when he told me that my father knew what he'd done, that he was sorry, and that he did love me. I saw that, along with the anger, hatred, and fear, there was a deep longing to be loved and not abandoned by him, a desire for a relationship with him—even though I couldn't have it. Hearing this was healing; it meant everything to me. When we left, I was no longer haunted by my father."

Sandy concurred. "I knew he wasn't capable and that it wasn't my fault," she said. This pilgrimage allowed her to stop running ("I think I was running from him," she had observed) and to flourish in a home of her own.

What Linda learned about her father helped her see her own life in a new light, and to take action to change it. "I realized the power in my own marriage was inequitable—I'd been looking for a father replacement. My husband also has a drinking problem, like he had. So I gave him an ultimatum, and told him that we have to go into counseling, that he has to change or I'll leave. I didn't believe I had that option before. I'm not paralyzed anymore." Both sisters left the funeral home feeling wiser and more powerful than when they had arrived.

Re-Visions

The Deathspace is a place of seismic movement. Truly terrible parents lose their power there. Children whose mothers or fathers were guilty of more routine crimes of the heart feel sympathetic and even come to identify with them. Flawed parents are discovered to have hidden virtues and idealized ones to have serious flaws. Family dynamics among the living—siblings and surviving parents—rearrange themselves like tectonic plates; alliances shift, fissures emerge.

Adults frequently speak of even extremely trying deceased parents in a bittersweet, elegiac tone that reflects a changed relationship. Beth Grant described how she disentangled herself from her mother and relieved the cycle of guilt and recrimination that paralyzed her as a younger woman. "Death's the final disconnect. It's harder to let go of a living human being who's clinging to you than somebody who's dead and only depressed in your dreams. From this distance I can see my mother with more compassion. I no longer blame her that I'm not married—I actually feel sorry for her. Her life had so much sadness; she didn't choose to ruin mine."

Jane Greenberg, the ex-fairy-tale princess, forgave her self-absorbed father, the producer. "In retrospect it's easier to see him as this guy walking around with his own damage, a victim of what we're all victim of," she said. "I feel a lot of compassion for this Class-A textbook narcissist."

James Marks, a sixty-four-year-old architect who had been haunted by parricidal fantasies, felt unexpected acceptance of his cruel father twenty-six years after his death. "As you get more understanding of yourself and the human condition in general, the judging piece falls away even when there's been a lot of pain," he said.

Wendy Hawkins, a fifty-four-year-old college administrator whose mother was alternatively manic or suicidally depressed most of the time, spoke of simultaneously appreciating her and recognizing how disturbing it was to grow up with her. "I've come to accept my mother with all her shortcomings and to see things about her I really love," she said twelve years later. Wendy was surprised how appealing her mother's wardrobe, flamboyant bordering on the bizarre, now seemed, although it had embarrassed her as a teenager. "It's funny—the things you couldn't stand are the things you miss." Losing this vibrant but oppressive presence inspired Wendy to appreciate the world more. "Her death gives my life a certain depth and makes me feel that I really must seize the day. I used to have a problem enjoying myself, but now I'm intensely aware I'm not going to live forever, either." As Jane Greenberg says, "The rage melts out of us."

In death, parental qualities that sons and daughters failed to recognize become salient; virtues that are lost on the young are appreciated by the middle-aged. Steadfastness in particular is not something children understand; they don't yet know how hard it is to sustain. Acting responsibly may not be glamorous, but it matters in the end. What was good and true finally comes through when the inevitable disappointment, like the rage, melts away—particularly if you work to make it happen.

Maggie Brown, whose father's premature death inspired her to stop smoking, originally shared her snobbish mother's opinion that he was an unsophisticated "Russian peasant." Even though Maggie remembered him fondly as a "warm, powerful, take-charge guy," and her "protector" as a girl, she also blamed him for the "foolish pride" and poor judgment that led him to dissolve a partnership in a way that seriously affected the family's finances. "It took me years to get over my anger at him for making such stupid choices and for taking care of everybody else but his family," she said. But as he aged, Mr. Brown's dependability and concern for others came to the fore. "My father used to visit every widow in their senior housing community daily to see if she needed anything. A thousand people came to his funeral; they had to set up loudspeakers in the parking lot," his daughter recalled, deeply impressed.

After her father died, Maggie "identified with his strength" and showed it by behaving similarly. "I made a promise to him in his coffin that I would assume his role as the protector of my mother," she said, and she made good on her promise. Using the same words to describe herself as she had used to characterize him, she said, "I took charge of all her affairs; I knew he would approve." When her mother told her that she "was just like my father," Maggie considered it a high compliment. She embraced the parental role so passionately that her mother, now in the late stage of dementia and utterly dependent on her, calls her "Momma."

Dennis Morrison, the language teacher turned novelist, had even more to overcome before he willingly took his father's place; he progressed from wanting to kill the man who had tormented and humiliated him early on, to emulating the "almost saintly" figure he cherished at the end. After time and suffering mellowed Dennis's father, his son was able to discern and then to incorporate the sterling character traits that their mutual fury had obscured. "His main characteristic was his sense of responsibility and loyalty. I've taken over my mother's care and finances from him. I'm becoming my father," he proclaimed proudly.

Even parental qualities that a child always noticed look different in retrospect; their meanings change. Diligence and doing one's duty, in particular, seem admirable and mature rather than stultifying when seen through adult eyes.

Bill Marshall was a thirty-year-old roadie touring with rock bands—he described himself as "an overage adolescent"—when his father, a hardworking orthodontist, died at age sixty-four. The "enthusiastically bohemian existence" Bill chose ("I never wanted a straight job," he told me) was as far away as he could get from the "terrifying boredom of the normal life" he thought his father was stuck in. "I sensed a lot of frustration in him; he treated every patient who walked in the door as his boss," Bill explained. But somehow his father's death galvanized him to reconsider both their lives. "When he died, I saw that it was time for me to tie up loose ends; that level of seriousness was not there for me. I'd never known how much I respected him—I was so grateful that I appreciated it in time to thank him, to say lots of things others don't get a chance to say."

Death made a man out of Bill. "His death made me less self-indulgent and less tolerant of nonsense. I became more demanding of others, more unwilling to endure frat-boy behavior, like ducking out on bills, from people I knew." Bill also became more demanding of himself, and proud to be so. "Aimlessness was no longer an option, and the time for reckless behavior had passed. I started taking better care of myself—working out, watching my diet more, and becoming a little more cautious in my associations. I settled in Dallas for some semblance of normality." There he took a regular job as a technician at a television station and started to live a more settled, steady life—the very existence he had dreaded and fled and that his father had epitomized. He found that it agreed with him. "I'd always feared that my life would mousetrap on me into routine, and I'm gratified that it didn't happen. I have a life of my own, a late coming-of-age, and new confidence. Only the luckiest of us turns into our parents," Bill concluded. He was lucky to discover he had a parent worth turning into.

The thoughts and feelings of offspring aren't the only things that change in the Deathspace; so do the dynamics of the entire family. Survivors discover one another when an undermining, disruptive, or overwhelming parent no longer interferes—and families that were held together primarily by obligation or by a parent's force of personality fall apart. Either scenario is liberating.

"Family gatherings are a whole lot easier now that my mother's not there," admitted Alice Gerard, whose mother had denied that her older brother had molested her and her younger brother. "Her influence was a big fog, oppressive over everything; it cleared when she died. We could look at each other and say, 'This is you.' People found their balance; all of us could talk. It freed us to tell the truth."

"My father's death signaled a new era," said James Marks. "Everybody enjoyed each other more. He'd been a millstone around our necks." Relationships between brothers and sisters often improve; James also said that his father's demise "created an opportunity for my brother and me to try to be closer."

But caring for sick and dying parents—and settling their estates—also sunders siblings, especially if there were fissures to begin with. Marsha Montgomery, the woman who moved to Rome after both her parents died, decided to sever her relationship with her brother because of the way he behaved when their father was ill. Ever the caretaker, Marsha built an addition to her house so that her difficult father could live there when his health deteriorated. For five years she cared for him and worked full-time simultaneously, at great emotional cost to herself and to her husband. "My brother was always too busy to see him, even though he lived a short flight away," she said. "The only time he made the trip he left two days later, saying it was 'just too depressing' to be there. He'd stayed with my father for one hour. Yet after my father's death he had the nerve to say, 'You didn't really do anything for him—you just hired a nurse.' I hated him for that; he made me feel horribly judged. We haven't spoken since. I knew I had kept the relationship going for my mother's sake; she had a falling-out with her own brother, and it was important to her that we get along. But I've never really liked him. Now if I saw him on the street I'd turn away." Blood may be thicker than water; sometimes it is more toxic as well.

The loss of a parent gives a child a priceless opportunity to reassess and to reexperience the living—self, siblings, and the surviving parent—as well as the dead. Necessary losses, bittersweet gains, and insights both touching and terrible happen in the hallowed ground of the Deathspace.

Joe Bailey not only recovered his faith when his mother died; he also discovered his father: "In a funny way my mother's death made it possible for my father and me to connect on an entirely different level. He was finally allowed to enter her territory—the more expressive, more emotional side; she cleared a space for us to have a relationship. Even the physical manifestation changed. He hadn't hugged me growing up, but then a real intimacy developed between us. After she died, each discovered in the other far more dimensions of personality than we'd imagined before. I'd never have known my father as I did in last seven years of his life if my mother had still been alive." Her loss transformed him, body and soul.

Peter Sawyer did not get close to his mother after his father died, but he did become her son. "My mother stopped husbandizing me—she just started acting like a mother," he said. "I'm comfortable with her now, as I am with my friends, in a way I haven't been since I was a kid. I like her, actually; I enjoy going to visit her. We have the same sense of humor, and there's no judgment. Both of us realize the freedom we have because he's gone."

The death of playwright David Schwartz's compelling mother brought his low-key father into the foreground in a disturbing, but enlightening, way. "All I ever thought was wrong with him was his absence; I didn't understand the potent negative presence that went into that absence. Her death expanded my awareness of the pathology of my father, and of my brother, who is just like my father." He learned that a passive parent is a subtly but seriously abandoning one.

~∞~

Sometimes a parent can only speak to you from the Deathspace—and sometimes you can only stop listening when you get there. Sasha Waldman, a thirty-nine-year-old jewelry designer, is convinced that her mother's death saved her life in an unusual way; it freed her from her still-living father. She came to the shocking, and ultimately self-preservative, conclusion that he neither loved her nor wished her well.

I met this tall, striking young woman at a mutual friend's party six months after our phone interview. She exuded intelligence and charm and was surrounded by a circle of men. It was hard to believe the ordeal she had endured in the three years since her mother died after a protracted battle with cancer.

Sasha had premonitions of her father's heartlessness during her mother's illness—the dying woman had wanted to spend her final days at home, and even with full-time nursing care he had refused to allow it—but nothing prepared her for his behavior at her mother's shivah, the Jewish week of mourning when friends and relatives visit the family to offer condolences. "He went around asking people to introduce him to women! Three weeks after she died, he announced he'd 'started a new chapter,' got remarried, and sold our family home, leaving only two boxes of mementos for me—nothing I would have chosen for myself—in the empty shell. My two older brothers and I were dumbfounded." Sasha tried to be sympathetic and supportive to her father ("he was alone and he couldn't even boil water") long after her brothers cut him off, until an episode six months later that she called "the last straw": "My father was talking to someone on his cell phone and it accidentally dialed my number and the conversation got taped. I heard him say that he disliked his children, that we were all worthless; I was devastated. When I made a copy and played it for him, he denied that the voice was his." Then she severed contact for good.

It took Sasha two years of intensive therapy to get over the blow and to unearth the real story of her parents' marriage and her own role in a family that looked good but was built on lies. "My mother got breast cancer when I was a teenager, and I grew up quickly," she told me. "Our relationship gave the appearance that we were close and friendly, but in fact I was her parent and caretaker." What she discovered about her father was far worse; checkbooks revealed that he had not worked for years and that her mother's parents had supported the family. "When I learned the history I couldn't imagine why she stayed with him. Now I look back and see all the patterns. It's been both painful and positive, my enlightenment about what kind of childhood I really had. My parents cared about themselves more than about us; their devotion was mostly a sham." Her father especially saw his talented children as "trophies." "I was just an image, a reflection for him. It was all about status that we achieved for his glory—his sons the doctor and the lawyer and his daughter the artist." Sasha realized that she had been an emotional orphan all her life. "In the truest sense I don't have parents and never did," she said.

It also became clear to her why she had never been able to have a relationship with a man. "As the youngest child and the only unmarried one, I was at their beck and call, sacrificing my own life. They liked the fact that I was single; it meant I was available to do things for them. It was always Sasha to the rescue."

Her father's behavior after her mother's death revealed his true colors and allowed Sasha to rescue herself. "I was not able to grasp any of this while my mother was living. If she hadn't died I'd have been the spinster daughter for the rest of my life. I'd be alone and never have sex again—without ever knowing that anything was wrong."

Although Sasha is delighted with her spectacular benefits, she still can't help worrying what other people will think; her experience is actually more common than she knows. "Two years ago I wouldn't have said anything positive came from it; I needed that long just to sort things out. Life's opened up for me—but it takes a special person to understand and not be shocked to hear me say so. I emerged having a self; it's an amazing gift. Death was the catalyst."

Self-Knowledge: The Ultimate Death Benefit

"It's not about me-me-me" is an insight—perhaps the most profound of them all—that being in the Deathspace facilitates; this was Jan Kahn's conclusion when she finally understood the roots of her late mother's devastating behavior. Some fortunate people figure it out during their parents' lifetime, but many more are only able to do so afterward. Empathy, sympathy, appreciation, and pity become easier to feel; you can walk in their shoes more comfortably when the owners no longer occupy them. Although recovering what was good in any parent (providing there is some to find) enriches life immeasurably, the greatest value in healthy detachment is that it is the best cure for victimhood. Discarding the role of passive sufferer activates a sense of control. To discover, at any age, that you are master of your fate—"of how extraordinary or pedestrian my life is," as Marsha Montgomery put it—is as thrilling as it is daunting.

Judith Thompson, a fifty-four-year-old musician and home health aid with a classic Brooklyn accent and a forthright simplicity of manner, had nightmares about her mother all her life. "She was always trying to kill me with knives or screaming furiously at me and hitting me. I'd wake up in a cold sweat. It felt like I was literally doing battle with her in my own body," she recalled. Then, two weeks before we spoke, as the second anniversary of her mother's death approached, Judith had a "light and welcome" dream about her for the first time: "I was sitting on the curb talking to my mother. She was asking my advice. I felt so happy, pleased, and surprised that I could be helpful, and I wasn't afraid I was going to give her the wrong answer. It was a sunny day."

Judith's progress from darkness to light, from being her mother's enemy in life to her trusted adviser in death, and from fear to confidence in herself, showed that she had changed inside and out. Stepping into her deceased mother's role as her father's caretaker, and virtual servant, opened her eyes. "It's like unraveling a very tangled ball of yarn," she said. "As I see his increasing demands, I think, 'Holy shit!' I was putting all of this on her. I see how manipulative my father is, how rigid and thoughtless he is, and how he blamed her for everything. This is the reason she was furious, and why I was so scared of her. She was cowed by him and enraged with him; she had to shut down because she couldn't bear it. She wanted me to make her happy, and hated me when I couldn't do it. I never knew her as happy, only angry, and I always felt bad because I thought I was responsible for her happiness. Now I understand why she was the way she was."

For a discontented parent to expect a child to fix her life and for that child to accept the impossible assignment is a common scenario, even though Judith's mother's vengeance was unusually fierce. But miserable firsthand experience taught Judith what her mother had endured; she didn't have to imagine it, as most of us do. She knew what it was like to be tyrannized by her father because she herself now bore the brunt of his impossible demands. "Now I rightly put blame—if that's really what it is—on him," she said.

Understanding why her mother "was the way she was" did not make her a candidate for sainthood in her daughter's eyes, but it did make her more sympathetic. The adversary Judith had demonized and considered the source of her own problems turned out to be just a desperate woman battered by life. Judith was particularly touched when she discovered a diary entry her mother had written as a lively adolescent ("Oh Life, please bring me happiness," it said); here was "a good side I didn't see before"—something to be inspired by rather than to dread.

Judith's first non-nightmare showed that the mother/daughter relationship that had eluded her in life was now hers. "One of the best things that's happened is that I'm making friends with her through the veil," Judith said. "I always used to be afraid of her, though it makes me sad to say so. I wish I could tell her. I think of her and I share things with her as if she is alive; she could be sitting here as we speak, listening to me and agreeing with what I'm saying. I hope she is! I plead with her to help me make good decisions about my dad's care."

Judith's newborn goodwill (and perhaps the beginning of love) is built from equal parts empathy and absence. Echoing Anita Suarez's sentiments, she says, "Our relationship is defused now; she can't do anything to me. Now there's no need to fight back because there's nothing to fight. The bad parts died with her; they're not real anymore." As the bad parts died, the good parts were revealed, and Judith claimed them as her own. "She had so much energy. At eighty-nine she wanted to go back to work as a waitress though she didn't weigh any more than the trays; she gave me real backbone."

Judith's sunny dream signals something even more valuable than a truce with her mother: faith and confidence in herself. Fear of "giving the wrong answer" and crippling insecurity no longer define her. "I always felt her negative judgment hanging over me. I was never good enough; if I'd win the Nobel Prize she'd say, 'Why didn't you win some other Nobel Prize?' This attitude made me constrained and self-critical—but now I know that the criticism really came from me. My hands used to shake in piano auditions, almost like I had to humiliate myself. I know I'm talented—why torture myself and ruin that? If you hobble yourself, you can only move ahead when you see it has nothing to do with anybody else. Seeing her differently shows me that I'm the only one that can hold me back from now on." When she grasped why her mother beat her, she stopped beating herself.

Along with the hateful side of her mother, Judith buried her own hatred, her guilt, and her need for self-punishment. She knows that whether she gets the Nobel Prize or the booby prize is nobody's responsibility but hers, and it feels wonderful. In discovering her mother beyond the veil, she discovered the key to her own happiness.

The Deathspace offers you a panoramic lens. If you study the view carefully, you also find a mirror.

CHAPTER 13

In Their End Is My Beginning

Cultivating Death Benefits

ം✑

Every adult whose parents die is entitled to death benefits. They are your "deathrights," part of your legitimate inheritance. But not enough people collect them. Most of the obstacles to acquiring what I believe are the most precious gifts of maturity are put there by you—a good thing since what you created you can usually dismantle.

Guilt, fear, and assuming that death benefits either don't or shouldn't exist prevent survivors from pursuing and celebrating them. Many people think literal-mindedly that the only possible nonfinancial advantage—other than being liberated from a really awful mother or father—is relief that the parent's suffering is over or that the burdens of caretaking are finally lifted. Self-fulfilling prophecies like these define possibilities away and make them harder to identify even when they appear.

Two contradictory beliefs—the conviction that our parents' lives have little impact on us as adults, and that their deaths are nothing but a devastating loss—blind us to the growth potential inherent in orphanhood. A third, that we can have no control over how a parent's death affects us, or which of their character traits we perpetuate, makes any good effects simply a matter of luck rather than the fruit of conscious action. These attitudes prevent you from receiving the best of a parent's emotional legacy or overcoming the worst. They also impede you from truly knowing your parents as people—and the considerable part of yourself that embodies them. Profiting from a parent's demise is neither disloyal nor incompatible with grief. Any loving parent—including flawed ones like mine, or Iris Connor's depressed but well-wishing mother—would want nothing less for their child.

Cultivating and then reaping death benefits involves creating a receptive state of mind and then constructing your parent's history, taking a Psychological Inventory, and translating your discoveries into action. Of these, the Psychological Inventory has the most clearly defined steps. Ask yourself the following questions:

1. What (character traits/attitudes/assumptions/behaviors) did you get from your parent that you cherish and want to keep?
2. What did your parent have that you didn't get and that you regret missing?
3. What did you get from your parent that you want to get rid of?
4. What did you need that your parent didn't have and couldn't provide?

Systematically seeking death benefits is the best way to find them, and these procedures are the essential tools; it is a rare parent whose personality cannot be mined for something meaningful, even if only a bad example. Think which of their attributes you can make use of at whatever stage of life you are in; things of great value (my mother's way of meeting death, for example) may still await you. Spend time going through all the stuff on every level, and take stock on a regular basis, just as you clean out your closets or your drawers to make room for the new—tasks we all avoid but are always glad when we tackle.

Conscious effort and a receptive, inquiring attitude pay huge dividends. Try to grasp your parents' secrets and their flaws, but most of all their stories—who they were and why. If possible get information from other people; their friends, your siblings—anyone who knew them in ways you did not—can provide other perspectives. Of course, your own memories are invaluable. Often it is possible to reforge a relationship with even the most difficult parents posthumously, on your own terms at last. Should this prove to be impossible, it will then be an intentional choice based on real understanding, a resolution rather than an automatic repudiation.

Even if you missed out immediately afterward, it's never too late to reap death benefits because opportunities to reconsider your inheritance—based on your ongoing Psychological Inventory—always present themselves. Death anniversaries and birthdays (yours and your parents') are good times to act. Seek ways to establish posthumous communication via things that remind you of the parent and that evoke intense emotions; putting my own lenses in my mother's red frames was a potent physical and symbolic action for me, and going to swim school was another. Personal rituals, like the letter Anita Suarez wrote to her rejecting mother decades after she died, can be curative; if your parent was as toxic as hers, it may be necessary to do as she did and wait until you feel autonomous enough to engage without endangering yourself.

Several immigrants' children whom I interviewed made pilgrimages to their parents' homelands or studied their cultural heritage, and it increased their insight and sympathy. James Marks saw his forbidding mother differently when he went to the impoverished Italian village where she was born. He said, "A wave of emotion leapt from my chest as I walked through those streets; I identified with my mother and how stultifying she found it there—she was the only one of nine siblings to leave—and I understood a piece of her. I felt a deep connection to her, a loving attachment that wasn't there before." James had a similar reaction when he went to Germany to see where his violent father had escaped from. Similarly, Judith Thompson became deeply involved in Celtic studies in her successful attempt to meet her Irish mother "beyond the veil."

Doing something a parent loved—swimming, dancing, singing, worshipping, going to museums, volunteering at an animal shelter ("It's my tribute to my father; he was always very sentimental about animals, a trait of his I am happy to embrace," Bill Marshall told me)—allows you to empathize and share the times when they were their happiest or best selves. So does using personally meaningful possessions of theirs. A patient of mine recovered some of her mother's capacity to nurture by brewing tea in her teapot; the smell of fresh-ground coffee—even the whirring crunch my mother's old grinder makes when I use it—revives good memories of her making me breakfast. Insights will announce themselves if you seek evocative experiences of your own, and revealing dreams will come, as they did for me and for Joe Bailey, Beth Grant, and many others. When parents are physically gone, the only person you have to get through to is yourself; willingness to overcome resistance and anxiety and learn the truth will be rewarded. Connections established after death may even allow you to know them for the first time.

Be on the lookout for death benefits and for circumstances and people that can lead you to them, as my young swim coach Cari led me; they turn up in unexpected places. Not long after her mother died—the mother who hated her and who had to be forced to relate and speak to her after a stroke—Tammy Carter was asked to write a manual on occupational therapy with mute, severely disabled children. "I never wanted to be around children at all before, but I love them now. These are the ones nobody wants—gravely damaged, almost repulsive. I give them unconditional acceptance," she told me. Rehabilitating these tragic children retroactively repairs the bond between her own damaged mother and the rejected child she was herself—a parallel Tammy did not recognize until we discussed it. Similarly, the insight that she was no longer impeding her own career to spare her now-dead mother's feelings only occurred to my colleague Laura Reynolds during our interview.

After Sasha Waldman lost her mother and severed her relationship with her destructive father, she got close to her ninety-year-old maternal grandfather. "I originally did it out of duty—my mother asked me to take care of him—but it became something else. I talk to him every day, and it's my favorite part of the day. I got a loving father figure; my mother never had a relationship with him, and I'm fixing that for her, too. It also helps me understand my mother and the choices she made. I get ten times back what I give him," she said. In my own case, listening to my patients describe (often with astonishment) how their lives changed for the better after losing a parent opened my eyes to the possibility while my mother was still alive; their experiences inspired me to anticipate and plan for the same. Thinking about death benefits, and then looking for them, helps makes them manifest.

The biggest impediment to acquiring death benefits is the conviction that you don't deserve them. Paradoxically, adults whose relationships with their parents were the most problematic are the most plagued by survivor guilt and fear of disloyalty. Although some degree of guilt is natural and almost universal, the very survivors who ought to get the most relief are most likely to become depressed and to feel like monsters, as though admitting that they have been liberated would be sacrilegious. Why do their parents "haunt from beyond the grave," as one woman put it?

Many children whose dead parents failed them in serious ways cannot permit themselves to thrive; as if to unconsciously validate the way they were treated, they think they do not deserve "the good china"—a fulfilling life. They cling to parents who rejected them, making excuses ("She grew up in the Depression" is a common one—as though nobody who did so became generous and loving). They are victimized by ghosts. To live well and happily would shed a cold, damning light on their parents' characters and behavior; survivors would be forced to recognize the profound deprivations they suffered. They would have to mourn for what they should have had, a difficult task indeed, but an essential one. Misplaced, phobic loyalty protects them from facing the truth about the past—a truth that must be addressed to create a different future. If you discover that you feel, as many people do, that your dead parent "put a spell" on you, do not simply resign yourself to your fate. Question your conclusions and confront your assumptions as I did when I recognized that I was accepting as immutable fact things (my inconsolability, for example) that I would never accept about anybody else. Depriving yourself of benefits perpetuates the worst aspects of a damaging parent/child relationship and often requires therapeutic intervention to reverse.

Whether your parents are still alive or long gone, the time to begin seeking death benefits is now.

There are many routes to death benefits; writing this book was mine. Whether your own effort produces a book, a letter, a diary, a painting, a poem, a photograph, a video, or a blog, the process of creating something makes thoughts comprehensible and feelings concrete. Investigating my relationship with my mother on paper helped me organize it, grasp it, and profit from it. Reconsidering her was as exhilarating as it was excruciating and gave me more hope and insight than I have ever known.

Any adult seeking death benefits can replicate the process I followed. First, to cultivate my benefits, I put myself on alert; emotional attentiveness primed the pump and helped focus my attention, consciously and unconsciously. Then, to reap them, I went through the stuff both literally and symbolically, over and over again (five times at last counting), paying attention to the emotions the physical objects evoked in me, opening myself to memories, letting feelings wash over me uncensored. I tried to question every assumption I had about who my mother was and how she influenced me, from as objective a stance as I could. I tried to address the way I thought as well as what I thought about and resisted the temptation to believe that anything was "just the way it is." Then I tried to apply what I had learned, seeking opportunities to expose myself to curative experiences and relationships that I realized I needed. As a result, every time I wrote about my mother and her legacy I learned something, made a new connection, heard and saw things I had never noticed before. It was a concentrated state of revelation that I hope to perpetuate. Actively seeking death benefits creates a feedback loop of awareness, action, and memory that is always accessible—a level of attentiveness that will accompany you subliminally for the rest of your life.

I have condensed the process into a complex but manageable series of psychological and behavioral practices (Cultivating) leading to three steps (Reaping) that anyone can follow—and didn't realize the acronym they spelled out until afterward:

Four Practices to Cultivate Death Benefits

Motivate yourself to address your relationship with your parents, before their death if possible. To do so is no longer taboo; it is smart. This commitment prepares you to see them in a new light. Make a conscious decision to engage with all your memories and resolve to investigate your parents' personalities. Invest the necessary time and energy to take a comprehensive inventory of them physically and mentally, and of their legacy. Do not leave it to chance.

Anticipate that there will be death benefits to discover. Give yourself permission to seek them actively. Identify your natural resistance, anxiety, guilt, and fear. Psychic preparation teaches you how to talk to yourself about your parents and your relationship to them. It sensitizes you, relieves you, and facilitates the process. It creates an environment in which benefits can be recognized and grow.

Meditate. A receptive, nonjudgmental stance is conducive to identifying and to creating death benefits. Think systematically and with an open mind about the ways—both good and bad—in which you resemble and differ from your parents. Question your assumptions about what's unchangeable. Ask yourself how you perpetuate ways of thinking and behaving that characterized them and that limit your capacity to live and love.

Activate. Death benefits are in your hands. Resolve to take action to discard the bad and reinforce the good, to see your parents whole. Look for traits to be inspired by; even the most flawed parent usually has some. Then, in order to reap what you have cultivated, follow the steps below; one of them, the Psychological Inventory, has its own set of procedures that builds on your previous experience of having taken a physical inventory when you sorted through your parents' material possessions. Repeated as necessary, this comprehensive program will permit you to collect the benefits you are entitled to—to make use of the opportunities that life presents, and to come into your own as never before.

Three Steps to Reap Death Benefits

1. Construct a narrative of your parent's history as objectively as possible; write it down.
2. Conduct a Psychological Inventory (see p. 215) of your parent's character, determining in detail what to keep and what to discard.
3. Seek new experiences and relationships to support the changes you need to make.

❧

I've just begun cultivating and reaping death benefits; I intend to pursue them for the rest of my life, and to encourage others to do the same. I will continue to question my fears and my negative assumptions, my turning off and turning away when people I love disappoint me or when I disappoint myself. I will keep trying to notice and to understand my tendency to sink and to forget to learn from experience.

I will be on the lookout for ever more ways to identify and to separate, to understand my mother better as I age. I want to do both what she did and what she was unable to do. I appreciate that the more I think about it, the more I am able to conjure the inspiring best of this complicated woman and banish the destructive worst. To pledge myself not to let myself off the hook makes me proud, and I hope it will make me wiser. I will work to make this new way of thinking a habit, an ongoing internal dialogue that will continue to change me and my world. Following her example, I will try to live to my fullest capacity, until my final hour if I can, to make the most of her great gift to me, one that neutralizes much of the pain and fear she also caused me.

If I am truly lucky, I will discover what she pointed the way to: that in my own last moment of consciousness I, too, will experience the beautiful moment in time that she was privileged to see. I hope it is the final benefit her death bestows on me.

Your Prescription for Collecting Death Benefits

FOUR PRACTICES TO CULTIVATE DEATH BENEFITS

1. Motivate
2. Anticipate
3. Meditate
4. Activate (includes the Three Steps below*)

THREE STEPS TO REAP DEATH BENEFITS

1. Construct a narrative of your parent's history
2. Conduct a Psychological Inventory of your parent's character (includes the Four Questions below)
3. Seek experiences and relationships to create necessary changes

FOUR QUESTIONS FOR CONDUCTING YOUR PSYCHOLOGICAL INVENTORY

1. What did you get from your parent that you want to keep?
2. What did your parent have that you regret not getting?
3. What did you get from your parent that you want to discard?
4. What did you need that your parent couldn't provide?

Acknowledgments

I want to thank the people I interviewed and my patients for sharing their experiences so openly with me and teaching me about death benefits. I am indebted to my agent, Michelle Tessler, and my editor, Jo Ann Miller, for believing in me and giving me the opportunity to write this book. My research assistant, Jessica Brinkworth, was an enormous help. Pat Towers gave me encouragement when I needed it most. Special gratitude goes to Jim Basker, Michael Carlisle, Chantal Deeble-Jackson, Bobbie Gallagher, Cari Laughlin, Terry Laughlin, Lisa Kogan, Paul Russo, Nina Smiley, Richard Snow, Terry Teachout, Anastasia Toufexis, Harriet Wald, and, as always, my husband, Richard Brookhiser, for their generous support.

This book is dedicated to Linda Marshall, my mother's guardian angel, and my beloved friend, for helping me discover more death benefits than I ever thought possible.

Notes

Chapter 2

49   *"Fifty percent have lost both parents"*: Umberson, Deborah, *Death of a Parent: Transition to a New Adult Identity*. Cambridge: Cambridge University Press, 2003 p. 15.

50   *"11.6 million adults"*: Kerr, Rita, "Meanings Adult Daughters Attribute to a Parent's Death," *Western Journal of Nursing Research* 16 (4) (1994), 347.

52   *"When asked to visualize"*: Miriam Moss and Sidney Moss, "The Impact of Parental Death on Middle Aged Children," *Omega* 14, no. 1 (1983–1984): 72.

54   *"Freud . . . felt 'uprooted'"*: J. Masson, ed., *The Complete Letters of Sigmund Freud to Wilhelm Fliess* (Cambridge, Mass.: Harvard University Press, 1985).

54   *"He wrote to his closest friend"*: H. Lehmann, "Reflections on Freud's Reaction to the Death of his Mother," *Psychoanalysis Quarterly* 52 (1983): 237.

55   *Princess Maria:* Leo Tolstoy, *War and Peace*, trans. by Rosemary Edmonds (New York: Penguin Classics, 1957), 859.

55 *"In one study":* Lawrence Calhoun and Richard Tedeschi, "Positive Aspects of Critical Life Problems: Recollections of Grief," *Omega* 20, no. 4 (1989–1990): 269.

56 *"hiding in a psychiatric journal":* Max Cohen and Louis Lipton, "Spontaneous Remission of Schizophrenic Psychosis Following Maternal Death," *Psychiatric Quarterly* 24 (1950): 724.

57 *"In his 1917 essay":* Sigmund Freud, "Mourning and Melancholia," in *The Standard Edition of the Complete Psychological Works of Sigmund Freud*, vol. 14, ed. by J. Strachey (London: Hogarth Press, 1963).

58 *"A recent study of 220 bereaved adults":* Scarlach Andrew, "Factors Associated with Filial Grief Following Death of an Elderly Parent," *American Journal of Ortho* 6, no. 12 (April 1991): 311.

58 *"Another researcher found":* Dov Shmotkin, "Affective Bonds of Adult Children with Living Versus Deceased Parents," *Psychology and Aging* 14, no. 3 (1999): 478.

Chapter 7

122 *"Being 'born again'":* In Matthew 10:35 (King James Bible), Christ says, "For I am come to set a man at variance against his father, and the daughter against her mother."

Chapter 10

160 *"Research shows that babies":* Obituary of Marian Radke-Yarrow, by Dennis Hevesi, "Marian Radke-Yarrow, Child Psychology Researcher, Dies at 89," *New York Times*, May 23, 2007.

Index